AT THE GARDEN'S GATE

A Personal Guide to Self-Discovery in Growing a Sustainable Backyard Meadow, Working with Nature and the Land, Living the Wheel of Truths

Judith Dreyer, MS, BSN

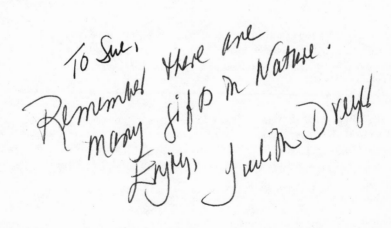

To Sue,
Remember there are
many gifts in Nature.
Enjoy, Judith Dreyer

█ FriesenPress

Suite 300 – 852 Fort Street
Victoria, BC, Canada V8W 1H8
www.friesenpress.com

Copyright © 2014 by Judith Dreyer, MS, BSN
First Edition — 2014

Cover design by Linda Silk Sviland

"The Gardener" by Martha Shaw

The content and stories in this book are meant to increase your knowledge of plants. The intent of the information presented is as a guide. Always practice caution when harvesting plants in nature. Check with three to five reliable sources for plant identification. Do not taste any plant in the wild that you do not know.

This information is in no way considered as a substitute for medical care, advice or treatment. Please consult your medical practitioners in the event of any medical concerns. The use of this book is at the reader's discretion. The author disclaims any liability directly or indirectly from the use of the information in this book.

ISBN
978-1-4602-5144-7 (Hardcover)
978-1-4602-5145-4 (Paperback)
978-1-4602-5146-1 (eBook)

1. Self-Help, Personal Growth, General

Distributed to the trade by The Ingram Book Company

REVIEWS FOR
AT THE GARDEN'S GATE

"At the Gardens Gate is a wonderful journey that includes the spiritual side of gardening and connecting with nature while at the same time giving you basic, helpful information on how to use plants to the best advantage. I highly recommend this book to anyone who wants to learn more about the plant world."
— Caryn Moya Block. award winning paranormal romance author

"Similar to the healing properties of the plants honored in its chapters, At the Garden's Gate enriches us through a shared botanical knowledge steeped with Native American teachings. A story which not only educates the mind, but the soul as well."
— Edward Bonapartian, author of The Stories of Our Lives.

"An inspiring and beautiful book, At the Garden's Gate, opens the door to our connection with the exuberant natural world of plants and herbs. Judith Dreyer's transformation of part of her lawn into a meadow, tracing the Native American medicine wheel onto her meadow, selecting common plants with extraordinary possibilities, brings us into the heart of how nature is always at hand to heal us physically and spiritually. How can we live our life enriched by nature's gifts that are within our easy grasp? Trained by L. Cota and herbalists, with echoes from Ayurveda and ancient therapies, Dreyer answers this question with vibrant examples from her nature apothecary. Consciousness of nature presences around her and their impact on her own personal reawakening from loss and change, this book invites us to embrace nature and renew ourselves."
— Pramila Venkateswaran, Author of Thirtha, Behind Dark Waters, Draw Me Inmost, and Trace.

TABLE OF CONTENTS

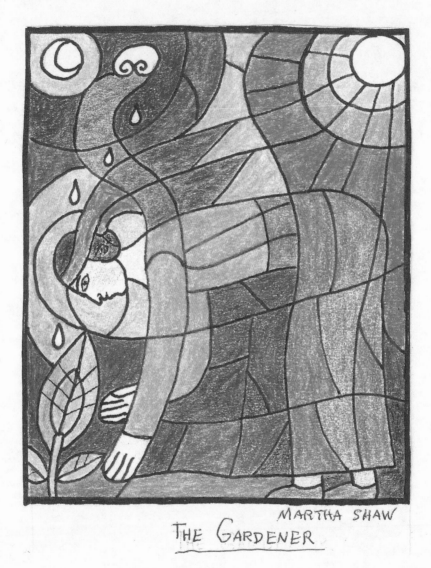

MARTHA SHAW

THE GARDENER

FOREWORD:
MAKA NUPA L COTA. (HUMAN BEING)

MANY YEARS AGO I MET THIS INCREDIBLE WOMAN, JUDITH DREYER, WHO CAME TO find her path among the Seneca people.

Some come and we know that they are not ready to walk the path of the connection to the spirit world. Some come and the elders watch them and guide them along the way. Judith was one of those who came and found her path into the beauty of the Spiritual World.

We each connect in our own ways for Creator has made us all unique.

Many times I would look out and see Judith sitting and watching the beauty of the day unfold. I knew in that moment she was destined to walk a trail of beauty. Each day she became calmer and more connected to spirit.

The Elders said that someday she would spread wisdom for sharing with many of her sisters and brothers.

I have been blessed to have walked with her through some of those times in her life that shaped and formed her into what she has become.

After many years of tribulations, and trials she has birthed this book of her journey to the center of the Medicine Wheel.

The day has finally come to share her wisdom with others so that the teachings may live.

In the pages of this book you will understand how simple it is to find your own roots and grow from them. The connection to all things will be shown to you. You will understand the beauty of the Mother Earth and all her creation.

Thank you Judith for being you, many heartfelt thanks from my old heart to yours. Maka Nupa L Cota. (Human Being, Cherokee and Lakota)

INTRODUCTION:
SIMPLICITY

"A garden should make you feel you've entered privileged space – a space not just set apart but reverberant – and it seems to me that, to achieve this, the gardener must put some kind of twist on the existing landscape, turn its prose into something nearer poetry."
—Michael Pollan, Second Nature: A Gardener's Education

THE PURPOSE OF THIS BOOK IS TO SHARE A STORY OF CHANGING A LAWN INTO A meadow, of personal growth during the time of co-creating with a land space, of walking a spiral path of inner seeking, of soul searching, and of sipping tea beneath the fragrant limbs of hemlocks while watching the sunset. This is also a book about turning a typical backyard lawn into meadowland, and about how meadows support wildlife, conserve resources, and protect our soil.

That we are a part of nature, just like the roots of plants and trees that intertwine deep into the forest soil, is a truth we have forgotten. Nature moves through her rhythms as we go about our day. A never-ending stream of movement, sometimes subtle or hidden from view, sometimes as strong as a rose's fragrance or a storm that kicks up and leaves debris when calmed, touches us. Poets and playwrights attempt to capture the heart of nature in words, stories, and songs that move and inspire us.

We find our way into our deepest selves when we let nature in, when we allow something to stir us to appreciate that which surrounds us.

Tea, a simple method of using plants in everyday life, has ancient roots. Teas, putting our plants in water, letting them steep for a bit, are often given to soothe. When prepared with knowledge and understanding of a plant's properties, teas foster healing of mind, body, and spirit.

This connection, the gifts of the natural world around us and our use of and relationship to this natural world, shapes us and our relationship to this planet and does so in mysterious patterns that call our soul.

My gardens began; as they began, my inner self stirred into seeking more. Step by step, season by season, I co-created and emerged into change while digging, planting, and allowing a meadow to form.

I am an avid reader. During my time with the meadow that is the subject of this book, I read so many books. I learned of the writing of many others who have written of their experiences with nature spirits (Devas), plant-beings filled with color and messages. These stories clouded the knowing of my own connection. [1]

During this period of reading and introspection, I found myself deeply drawn to Native American teachings of my ancestry – their approach to taking care of the land, their belief in how precious her resources are, and their practice of asking before taking. I wanted to know the spirits of earth, not from the books but from my own experiences. The practice of asking and giving thanks resonated inside me as I tended and harvested plants from this backyard meadow.

Seasons changed and I watched my yard spaces change and take differ- ent shapes and forms. During this time I dug out the roots of discontent. I weeded negative thoughts from my own thinking, and I blossomed slowly under the sun's light in a way I could not have imagined.

Every day, the wind moving through the leaves created an incessant chatter for the day's chores. Birds punctuated the melody with high notes and low as if playing a flute. Crows came in and provided an intermittent percussion. Bees buzzed, ever determined in their sweet unwavering task. Butterflies alit in such a way it seemed they were whispering to the flowers some secret, gossip, or tantalizing detail. Dragonflies hovered like helicop- ters, moving in a pattern special to them.

The simplicity of being with everyday movement, sound, cadence found in the meadow today feels extraordinary.

I learned of the cycles and began …

We have forgotten how to accept these endless cycles that carry the beat and pulse of the earth, a movement as constant as the rotation of the earth around the sun. The ancients taught that what is outside us is inside us. We are the earth and she is us. There is no separation.

The tremendous gift outside our doors is often taken for granted, abused, misunderstood.

Co-creative partnership is our journey, both the earth's and ours. This meadow taught me the value in completing simple daily tasks and mundane chores and the value in the uncomplicated acceptance of being.

Our great mystical teachers remind us over and over that we cannot control the future. The tasks performed in the now with awareness and inner understanding of our place and of our relationships, reap gifts that create our future.

My journey into the healing arts began with nursing. When my second child came around, we had health issues to deal with. His lack of foundational health pushed me to seek other systems of healing, something that would break his pattern of ear infections and antibiotic over-use.

I stepped off the Western medical model, the model of allopathy, with fear, uncertainty, and trepidation.[2] Slowly, I learned from Naturopathic physicians, chiropractors, and others, about a holistic point of view that was and still is foreign to Western medical practice and study (though today that is changing.)[3] Like the decision to watch a meadow bloom and change with the seasons, my progress into the idea of holistic health did not happen overnight. The acceptance of the idea that medicine and food could be found in common weeds, through the many resources of meadow and woods, was a journey.

As the lawn became a meadow, I became filled with firsthand knowledge of the nourishment plants offer to mind, body, and also spirit. Gradually my medicine chest became supplied with natural remedies and nontoxic cleaning products.

The change was more than simply a focus on medical solutions: I wanted to give my family foundational health, free not only of the dependency on synthetic drugs but also from the fumes of toxic cleaning products and residues of pesticides in unclean food. I bought organic when I could, shopped at local farm stands, and moved away from those products of an industrial model.

This period of time ended. I left that land in 2001. The meadow is now back to lawn, occupied by new owners who keep it mowed and tidy. I have moved to different places, opened and closed a health food store, and now teach holistic health at a university level. I took Master Gardener training from the local agriculture extension office. I found that despite the continued emphasis on pesticides and "control" of nature, that there is interest in rethinking our use of landscapes. Lawns are heavy consumers of resources. They consume tremendous amounts of synthetic fertilizers, pesticides, weed killers, gas, and water.

The Earth Institute at Columbia University states that today:

1. Lawns occupy some 30-40 million acres of land.

2. Lawnmowers account for 5 percent of the nation's air pollution.

3. 17 million+ gallons of fuel are spilled in refilling lawn and garden equipment. (This is more than the oil in the Valdez spill.)

4. Homeowners spend 10 times the amount of pesticide and fertilizers per acre on lawns than farmers do on crops.

5. The runoff from the above chemicals becomes a major source of water pollution.

6. 30 to 60 percent of urban fresh water is used on lawns; most of this is wasted due to poor timing and application.[4]

Universities such as Purdue suggest that modest changes in our use of lawn space can have big effects.

This book is born out of a desire to share one woman's journey from transforming a lawn into a meadow in suburbia, the changes that came with one acre, the variety of plants and critters that emerged, and in tandem, the care and the deep growth found in allowing myself to reconnect to nature. This journey took me through a gate of understanding and reconnecting, of partnering with nature that fulfilled a dream. The paths I literally created and the inner paths I chose to explore changed my perception of nature, how we can work with these presences and co-create with the earth. Today it seems the earth is calling us to change, to rethink our use of her gifts, to co-create with nature once again. And in the spirit of the great sages past and present, the time is now.

ROOTS: THE BEGINNING OF
MY WALK WITH GARDENS

I DON'T KNOW THE WHY OF "IT", JUST THAT "IT" SEEMED TO BE A SENSE OF WANTING, a yearning to take care of the earth in some measure. Of course how could I possibly know back then that the earth can take care of herself? That awareness did not come till much later. The feeling within me, the "it", took hold as I entered adulthood and began to explore the philosophical musings of the ways of the world.

In college, we were hopeful, sitting up till 2 a.m. singing folk songs. We never tired of filling the empty stairwells with words of hope, words of peace and "we shall overcome", because if we did, then it would be back to the books or worse – a feeling that maybe we could not change the world.

We were desperate in our conversations to find the "why". Why the fighting? The Vietnam War divided us as a country and seemed purposeless. Why the chemical contaminations? Dow Chemical came to campus to recruit students for jobs.

When they did, we asked about and protested against the use of napalm overseas, not only on foreigners but on our own soldiers. The Chicago Seven, the grape workers in California, women's rights, civil rights, grabbed headlines daily. We sang and discussed, debated till early morn. Why won't they listen to us? Who were/are "they" anyway?

College came and went. I earned a Bachelor of Science degree in Nursing, and before long I was working a 42-bed geriatric ward from 3 p.m. to 11 p.m. The guitar was put aside as I took art and dancing lessons before work. Vacation was reduced to two weeks per year. I remember the feeling my first year out of school and the panic that set in. "What? No semester break, no summer break?" This was the real world of paychecks and rent. At 22, I felt I was up to the task and welcomed the freedom to be on my own.

1

My first apartment had a little patio, and there I set up a couple of window boxes on stands that framed this outdoor space. Every day before work I would water them and admire the pinks and purples of never-ending petunia blooms that actually flowered throughout the summer with my simple tending. They were cherished. I think of this time as the time of the window boxes, an initiation of sorts in to the world of plants. Could I keep them alive and blooming with my schedule? Yes. I did. I appreciated the task of dead heading and watering, a daily ritual throughout summer months.

Three years later I moved to my next rental, a 100-year-old farmhouse, in the early autumn. I left geriatrics and got a job in Community Health Nursing, Visiting Nursing, or VNA for short. The farmhouse seemed ideal as the town was next to the city where I would be working. When I moved there in the fall, I had no idea of the beauty buried deep in flower beds around the house and the white picket fence that would burst into color the following spring.

That first spring brought a banner of color and a rhythm all its own. First came the purple crocus, emerging through New England snows. Next, when the snow and ice had melted and spring began to tease us with a bit of warmth, yellow and white daffodils came. Bright orange-red poppies took up the symphony as deep purple irises displayed their bearded petals. Peonies, planted with care in some earlier time, stole the show with their heady perfume and full blossoms – though maybe I am a bit biased. Then the hedge roses, with pastel color and fragrance, bloomed and bloomed.

Gorgeous petals in white and pink graced our tables for as long as they showed their flower faces on sturdy vines. I marked the days and the seasons of spring and summer by the flowers that bloomed in their perfect time.

In this place I took many a walk down a nearby country lane that followed a stream bed. I found a little book on wild flowers and was soon able to identify a few. Tall, airy Queen Ann's lace, prolific goldenrod, bright orange hawkweed, all common for sure, but at that time these were new acquaintances.

One day as I walked by the stream bed, I found wild onion, an edible. I took some home and made a stir-fry with them; strong, pungent, and woodsy in flavor, in no way sweet and familiar like the store-bought onions.

Something pecked at me inside, but I had no idea what the feeling was. I viewed myself as an ordinary woman finding peace from a hectic nursing career. Walking by roadside wildflowers and observing flowerbed gardens started decades prior proved soothing.

Some roots go deep. Some seeds can stay buried for 100 years until a bit of sunlight finds them.

During this time I was content to gather and fill vases, admiring the textures and scents, and was content to enjoy their presence and beauty in and around my home. Somehow, watching the progression of each flower's cycle of growth, bloom, and decay, seemed to cradle a sense of something more in nature – something that seemed mysterious.

Here, in this country farmhouse and in the nearby lanes, my love of wild flowers took root. Bouquets of many common plants and their leaves filled vases for the three years I lived here. I hardly knew what food they required or if any fussing. I simply oohed and awed over them. I picked some for the house and enjoyed them. Inside and outside, I loved the soft fragrance of roses and peonies. I loved the colors and shapes mixed with various greens selected from the meadow's abundant fronds. It became a weekly ritual to fill vases and then empty them, only to repeat the cycle and fill them again as one flower faded and another one bloomed.

During my years here, autumn would bring a sadness that the beauty and grace of summer was ending. I watched plant after plant follow their own unique path of coming and going, much like my patients who graced me with their uniqueness. They too had color, high notes and low; personalities that gave me an insight into life's hard times and soft times.

The famous passage in Ecclesiastes states that everything and everyone has a season, "a time to die and a time to be born." During my three years at this farmhouse, I picked up the guitar again and revisited old folksongs when I could. Strumming my way into the melodies of love and restlessness, of hope and travails, helped me glimpse life just a little bit more. Like roots that grow deeply and gather sustenance, I stored my feelings of restlessness and hope deep within me. Wanting more, I began a garden of my own: Vegetables this time; a need to supply food, preserve food, to store food so our larder would be full.

In this old farmhouse, I fell in love, I married, and three years later, moved away.

That became the pattern of my life: I moved from this farmhouse, married, moved again and had children. I put in window boxes and gardens where I could.

After moving a couple of times, we settled in southwestern Connecticut. It is here in this typical suburban home that my story takes form. I began to plant and to dig the earth for a garden. I started with vegetables. I filled the freezer with its harvest; tomato sauce made from scratch, adding green beans, peppers, and seasonings. We ate the rest in summer salads as the garden produced. Marigolds, zinnias, cosmos, and wild daisies created a border.

My vegetables would look beautiful the first few weeks after planting, and then we would go away one week or two in July, which was and is the peak time for New England gardens, especially for vegetables. Inevitably, I'd come home to sorry looking plants, wilted, bug infested, that no amount of water and sunshine or apologies seemed to revive.

A year after we moved to Connecticut, I became aware of a special event, the harmonic convergence that occurred in August of 1987. I became intrigued with the Mayan calendar, Hopi prophesies and dreams.[5] My dream gates opened, and I had incredible dreams and inner urgings to learn more about self and about the earth. During the next three years I read voraciously about Native American philosophy and found myself wanting a teacher. I also found an herbalist who knew a bit of Native American philosophy and their relationship to plants. I attended my first herbal class and began to revisit my backyard; at least I began to wonder what was growing in between blades of grass.

I also noticed that the grass that we had mowed towards the back of the property contained common weeds that were edible and had medicinal properties. I learned to identify them one by one and became excited. My husband at the time went along with my ideas, and we let the grass grow to see what would come up. What plants and wildflowers would bloom?

What plants could I use for colds and coughs? What plants were actually growing here?

After a couple of years passed I brought in purple coneflower. Then someone gave me comfrey root cuttings. Nettles were planted near the compost pile. Mugwort stayed on the garden's perimeter (though this shrub relentlessly traveled inside). Evening primrose and spearmint thrived outside the fence. Eventually yarrow, butterfly weed, wild daisies, lavender, sage occupied the interior. Dandelions and lamb's quarters prospered inside. Some consider them weeds. They showed up naturally, and I set out to learn about their edible properties. I appreciated their arrival and felt it important to let them stay. As a co-creative partner, some weeds did and do go, get added to the compost pile. Some were food sources and were left, which doesn't always create a pretty garden. Weeding, harvesting, and pruning are expected activities when we co-partner with nature.

My gardens shifted and changed and captured the attention of numerous bee species that hummed incessantly on hot August days. Butterflies covered the purple coneflowers, adding oranges and blues to the palette. Dragonflies flitted, often landing on my arm or sleeve while I would marvel at their varied colors.

During this period of transformation, I began to love the meadow and her gifts. I became a steward, allowing nature's hand to emerge in the yard while adding some of my favorites. Seeds sprouted on their own. Plants emerged without my interference. All that came, all the colors of the meadowland, entranced. I was hooked. In this small meadow, I found my place.

In this transition from lawn to meadow, I looked at myself as a partner with nature. Over several years and with care, I began to arrange the meadow area and the smaller gardens. On the right side of the property back by the tree line, I began with a twenty-five by thirty foot space where we mowed a small circle in the center. Here I felt guided to consider the circle as a medicine wheel. From the outer edges of this space we mowed four paths into the center, each one following one of the four directions. The journey I had undertaken into Native American culture up to this point inspired me to create this wheel within the meadow, to somehow have a place to come to, to honor the earth teachings I was gathering in.

When life imposed on my serenity I would often sit here in this center, determined to find answers. I used the medicine wheel that I dreamed about and read about and then created as my focal point. The four directions – North, South, East, West – became a part of me and gave me a sense of direction.

Now don't laugh at the pun here for no pun was intended. I was serious. Wheels are found all over the earth. Some of the Native American elders I met along the way shared their understandings of the wheel.[6] They stressed over and over to sit in the silence and wait for the answers to come. "Patience, my friend," they would say. "Go sit and allow your dreams to speak to you."

The way of spirit is simple. Our divine guidance does not come in long dialogues. As I weeded between medicinal plants in the formal gardens, hot, sweaty and asking "why" again, I would hear on a rare occasion a voice, soft as the wind but just as distinct, answer me.

"Cycles."

That was all. Nothing more or less, as I struggled with the day's frustrations while weeding. One word I have never forgotten. Sometimes I would feel a sense of love, a knowing that I was not alone outside doing simple chores. This time I treasured.

As the meadow and gardens developed, birds and bees, other critters patrolled the meadow and created a vibrancy. Any disturbed soil brought surprises. We put in a pool, and the soil removed from one area was left beneath a strand of hemlocks. The next spring coltsfoot put up little yellow flowers, a new plant for me to get to know. Did you know that a coltsfoot flower resembles the flower of a dandelion? And that they both pop out around the same time? This occurrence highlights the need for correct plant identification. After the flower wanes, deep silvery green waxy leaves in the shape of a coltsfoot take their place till fall arrives. Wild roses flourished in the meadow, especially with periodic haircuts.

I soon realized I only had to set up the space and gently prod or add a plant here and there, and nature did the rest! Wild flowers didn't need me to fuss; well maybe they needed me to shape the space and prune a bit, but they are hardy and prolific. I didn't have to measure fertilizer or worry about infestations. The plants helped each other out, and I noticed they helped the vegetable garden too, companions in the true sense of the word. This lawn space was turned into a meadow with small, more cultivated, gardens nearby. The meadow produced flowers and grasses all on its own. I could harvest and gather and make herbal products from this bounty. I felt I was in partnership here. I felt I was working with nature, following the cues and messages she sent.

At the same time I sculpted a wheel with paths in the four directions on the right side of the meadow area, we put in a spiral path on the left side, a twenty-five by thirty foot area. This became a meditation path of double spirals. During two springs, a formidable spider became the gate-keeper of this spiral path created for quiet time. She wove an incredible web that I gave thanks for everyday as I passed her way. She literally positioned her patrolling at the beginning of the path, and one could not help but notice her black with a yellow-patterned body as she sat in the center of her web. I would walk by with care and respect, hoping that she trusted me to not disturb her silken web. Her web sat about a foot off the ground in the sun. I since learned she was probably a black yellow garden spider *(Argiope aurantia)*

You have no idea what a feat of courage this was for me. As a child, I would scream and nearly lock myself in frozen fear if a spider dared come nearby, and I worked diligently up to this point in my life on releasing and reducing my fear of spiders. This spider and my daily passage by her web marked a new part of my journey.

She taught me that the web of life is not straight or linear. Life weaves a path and one follows. I followed my heart and created this meadow with nature. Much like a new shoot that grabs the sunshine and grows, I too grew and changed, while bearing witness to the growth before me.

When we moved to Connecticut in 1986, I had stopped working at this point and had become active in various organizations in town through my son's activities. We were a multicultural town, and we had to get along. If we helped each other, the activities flowed smoothly. When egos and tempers flared, we lost a bit of our sense of community. The modern world is tough with the merging of cultures and the breakup of families.

How can we live side by side treasuring our roots, when we don't stay long enough to grow them? How can we blossom in new land? Are we hardy enough to be transplanted? Will we be seen as just another weed, a focus of annihilation?

The meadow became my teacher and I, the student. Over time, the meadow became a haven for wildlife. The thorny stems of wild roses gave shelter and safe harbor to rabbits and sparrows, cardinals and finches. Hawks and crows flew overhead hunting for dinner. Skunks came out at night, nosing the ground as they ate the grubs in the grasses. Deer munched without hesitation and allowed me to sit in a hemlock grove nearby and bear witness to their passing. Coyotes came by too, though I rarely caught a bushy tail at the forest's edge. Summer evening stars shone above while fireflies twinkled and teased in the waning light. At dusk, the bats would begin their flights, their dark wings glimpsed momentarily here and there.

When darkness would begin to fall, my dog, Foster, and I would often go outside. We would sit, watching the moon rise and fall, casting its shadows deep into the grasses. During these times, I learned to sit quietly without expectation, a lesson in patience that fed my roots and nourished growth occurring without my awareness.

I was and am a nurse, and I wanted to help others. Which plants could we eat? Which plants could provide medicine? These became my mantras. I decided to study herbology, the art and the science. My Native American elder friends reminded me that everything we need is beneath our feet.

Little did I know how my enchantment with my meadow would grow and nurture a love for the earth. The "it" I felt stirred within again. As life unfolded, "it" began to take on a form, and this meadow, sweet and present, and the plants under my feet, became my focus for nearly twelve years.

STEMS: CREATING STRUCTURE, GRATITUDE, INTENTION, AND RITUAL

Do everything with an attitude of gratitude.
—Grandmother Kitty, Nakota Sioux, 1925-1994

APPRECIATE, GIVE THANKS, BE GRATEFUL, WORDS FOR ALIGNING TO A HIGHER purpose and power. Grandmother Kitty spoke these words often in our many gatherings. Many others today write and speak on the benefits of living our lives gratefully. Gratitude enables us to claim ourselves differently too, for when we are grateful, we have an opportunity to acknowledge both the mundane and the holy.

The easy part is to be grateful for what "we" have in the outside world, not only material things, but also those human and natural resources found in home, family, and job. What is harder is to be grateful for those circumstances that have shaped us. It's easy to be grateful for the new car or job we've been wanting. But, can we be grateful for the person or event that seemed to bring hardship? Can we find the teaching, the nugget of truth in a difficult situation that shaped us and be grateful? It is one of the challenges of our human experience.

Work in the garden is intentional, and ritual brings us into partnership with nature. Weeding, sifting soil, digging up the roots of a tree stump, planting, getting sweaty and dirty, dealing with pesky bugs, all these activities make us a part of the process of nature.

As in the garden so in the soul. Negativity can be weeded out. Sweating we cleanse. Water purifies. Activity keeps muscles strong. Working around other creatures reminds us we are not the only species. And in the process, we can compost the hurts, regrets, and disappointments into something beautiful.

All humans live by seasons and cycles. This place earth, that we call home, is governed by those, and we are as well. Grandmother Kitty, an elder I sat with and met at the first women's council I attended at the Seneca Wolf Clan, Cattaraugus Reservation in New York, often spoke of the indigenous tribes here, the Americas, the Aboriginals from Australia, or the Maoris from New Zealand, for example, that recognized the rhythm of nature. The earth's seasons are woven in stories and mythologies of those cultures shared today and into day-to-day life. My study of other medical models such as Ayurveda from India and Traditional Chinese Medicine, or Tibetan, all speak of the world of nature and the important connection to the earth's elements and seasons for health, for food production, for medicine making, for community. In essence we, the human as the microcosm, are a reflection of the outer world, the macrocosm. So therefore the elements, the seasons, the cycles that govern nature govern all of us.

Part of the reason I am sharing my story is to convey something to you of the presences that are a part of our world. Often unseen, these presences have been ignored, disavowed, made fun of, cast off as demons, generally debunked as myth in the relentless Western pursuit of the scientific approach. In this world of "hard reality", if we cannot see or know or measure a "nature spirit", we assume this realm does not exist.

Native American culture, Celtic culture, Indian Ayurvedic teachings, Taoism, and other belief systems all offer a consistent acknowledgement of the forces of nature. Each season has characteristics that describe qualities of health, foods, and an element. Each season represents a life cycle. Farmers from around the world often govern their growing and harvesting practices by the cycles of the moon. Deciduous trees produce new leaves in spring, lose them in fall, and stand bare through winter.

In fact, more than sixty to seventy percent of cultures around the world believe in the power of other forces that cannot be felt, manipulated, or seen.

Call these forces Devas, Nature Spirits, wee folk, leprechauns, fairies, regardless, something seems to govern the life of plants, whether the tallest oak or the tiniest seed.

During my herbal studies I heard of a community called Findhorn, a place in Scotland that works directly with nature spirits in co-creating gardens. Begun in 1962 and continuing to today, this exceptional center attracts students and teachers from all over the world. Started as a small spiritual community funded by "faith that God will meets its needs if the community follows the esoteric laws of manifestation." They talk to the plants in the garden, and "the plants seems to like it so much that they respond by growing out of sand and blossoming in the snow."[7]

Findhorn's gardens attracted the attention of garden and horticultural professionals. Their communion with nature and their results were astounding, so much so that those of us stepping into the world of herbalism at the end of the 1980's found guidance and an understanding of nature beyond books. We weren't "crazy" in our love of the earth or in our sense of something more contained in those realms. Findhorn membership communed with Pan and Devas receiving direct guidance on how to co-create with nature that not only enhanced the human world but also enhanced their natural realms. In the act of sowing a garden, Findhorn found seeds of opening to a deeper consciousness. They fostered a sense of cooperation that opened many minds to the possibility of gardening in partnership with these spiritual presences.

It is hard for me to write this, to attempt to explain these presences to you. Our culture does not readily accept them yet our Hollywood and TV excites our imagination with any number of fantastic creatures – Pan, leprechauns, fairies, and trolls.

What I am writing about is real, as real as any essence of being. The reality of such is shown in the results at such a place as Findhorn.

Writer and gardener, Machaelle Small Wright's *Perelandra, Garden Workbook* provided an introduction into the world of Devas, Overlighting Devas, and Pan here in the US.[8] She informed me that these beings are part of the angelic realms that co-create with us in our landscapes and our place in the world.

Findhorn and Perelandra's direct communication and guidance from Pan and Devas helped me develop and persist in my intention to work with nature more deeply and to trust in that experience.

Adopting some of Wright's suggestions, combined with the teachings from my Native American elder friends, created a ritual format for me to follow. This format gave me a feeling of structure in working with nature out my back door. I added them to my daily life, specifically using a basic four-step process for my morning routine that anyone can follow. These are **gratitude, intention, ritual,** and then, **letting go.** The first and most important is the act of showing Gratitude.

1. **Gratitude**

Gratitude is defined as expressing appreciation.

When I committed to learning about edible and medicinal plants, two threads joined: the love of learning and the teachings of gratitude.

My Native American elders began each ceremony with prayers of gratitude to all of creation and to all our relations. Tobacco was offered; we were taught to give thanks and offer that thanks, using a pinch of tobacco, before taking from the plant kingdom. If one did not have tobacco, then we could spit or take one strand of hair and leave that as an offering.

I kept tobacco with my garden tools and by the back door. I made the commitment to give thanks when I started my day. I learned to ask permission before I began work in the garden and to even ask permission to enter when I ventured into other forests. Later on, I studied with a few elders from different tribes and learned that tobacco was considered masculine and corn meal feminine. I was taught to use tobacco in the morning facing east and cornmeal at night facing west, praying to the four directions, the four winds, each time.

I am personally drawn to Native American practices. They resonate deeply with me and are a part of my heritage, and these actions became my daily practice. I appreciated the consistency of routine, expressing gratitude and felt I was honoring the plant kingdom.

Each individual should find his or her own prayer and practice – that which works best for the individual. A colleague of mine often placed a small piece of chocolate on the ground in thanksgiving. It was her favorite food. Ultimately, it does not matter what words or substance we use, for I have come to believe it is our heart's sound that is heard.

2. Intention

Intention is defined as "an act or instance of determining mentally some action or result." Dr. Wayne Dyer, in his book *The Power of Intention*, suggests that, *"Intention is not something we do or acquire but something we connect to."*[9]

Stepping out the back door into my yard, I knew my intention was to connect with nature, to learn about the plants not just physically but to glean something of the plant kingdom's essence. It was also my intention to walk the ground with respect for all of life that lived, to honor "all my relations", a common phrase/concept in Native American circles. I repeated this intention as I took a pinch of tobacco into my hand.

3. Ritual

Ritual is defined as "an observance, an act, or action repeated regularly in a precise manner." From another perspective, Thomas Moore says this about ritual in his book, *Care of the Soul:*[10]

"Ritual maintains the world's holiness. Knowing that everything we do, no matter how simple, has a halo of imagination around it and can serve the soul it enriches life and makes the things around us more precious, more worthy of our protection and care. As in a dream a small object may assume significant meaning, so in a life that is animated with ritual there are no insignificant things."

Consistently showing up every day, using tobacco to carry my intention, saying my prayers to the four directions brought me to an awareness of meaning, of what some call "the work of the soul".

Earlier, I had for many reasons, left organized religion. As I learned more of my Native American heritage, my heart found the teachings of my ancestors more fulfilling. I learned to listen to inner guidance in a more consistent way. As I mentioned earlier, dream awareness is taught in the Native American culture but not in mainstream society. Nighttime dreams fostered and supported this growth, gave me a sense of the sacred and the Divine. Listening to this nighttime guidance and practicing a consistent daily ritual pulled me forward into learning more and more. Without conscious intent and without ritual, the foundation of learning would not have had the substance or fostered the deep connection to nature I have come to appreciate and value.

4. Letting Go

Letting go helps us to live in a more peaceful state of mind and helps restore our balance.
—*Melody Beattie, The Language of Letting Go*

I stepped into my backyard any morning I could or set up space in my home. I faced the East, took a pinch of tobacco, breathed deeply, and then silently stated my intention, my prayer for the day. I blew these intentions, prayers into the tobacco releasing them to the wind, to the ground, or a conch shell bowl, letting go of expectations.

I began most mornings this way. In accordance, I walked through my days and my nights accepting the routines before me. Inspirations, ideas percolated and then the ideas for paths in the meadow formed.

As I previously mentioned, a medicine wheel was shaped with a lawn mower. In an area about twenty feet by thirty feet to the right of the backyard in front of the tree line, I mowed four paths to the center of the space. Each path was placed and represented each of the four directions. After the medicine wheel was formed, I carefully cut a double spiral on the left. This became a meditation path in an area about twenty feet by thirty feet.

Gradually my enclosed garden took the shape of a figure eight, the symbol of infinity. After a couple of years in this location, we decided to put a pool in, a circle, closer to the house.

Symbols, paths, dreams all converged. During this time I had made a serious commitment and intention to learn about the world of dreams (which I will share in my next book) and was consistently documenting my dreams and learning from them. I felt none of this was an accident and felt in awe, honored to work this land, the gardens and meadow.

Gratitude and asking, setting intention, following a ritual pattern to begin and to tend the day, then letting go became my routine. Letting go is often the hardest when the stuff of life crowds in, yet this simple ritual taught me to trust. Life is mysterious. Working with unseen presences in nature is mysterious. In letting go, I learned to trust, have patience, observe, act with conscious awareness, or as some would say, with mindfulness.

In summary, to begin the process of connection, follow these actions:

1. Set your **intention.**

2. Express **gratitude** for all you have and know.

3. Do the above in a **ritual** fashion, consistently. Gather sage, feathers, rocks, pictures, and tobacco, whatever speaks to you. Keeping it simple always works.

4. **Let go** and let God, the Divine, receive that which you put out. No more, no less.

For those of you who are new to this, I invite you to take on these practices. The benefits are not necessarily tangible, but are no less or perhaps more powerful because of their intangible nature.

Those among us who commune with nature spirits know that we humans have really maligned this land and all kingdoms that reside here. Giving thanks, asking permission of something that contains divine order and essence, stating our intentions clearly can begin the process of healing our relationship with nature and ourselves. We are not inherently alien to Nature, but a part of her.

THE MEDICINE WHEEL

IMAGINE BEING BLIND AND BEING BORN ON AN "INDIAN" RESERVATION AT THE TURN of the century. Your oral tradition was taught and passed on to you without the aid of typewriters, phones, computers, or books. You grew up, had your family, and saw the world change so fast, you wondered if the way of your ancestors would be forgotten. You sat your grown daughter down and told her she would be the voice between two worlds, hers and that of the "boat people", the European white settlers who now dominated "Turtle Island" (America); those settlers who forced her ancestors off their land and onto reservations and whose generations since have struggled to keep their culture and traditions alive.

I met Grandmother Twylah Nitsch at the first Green Nations Herb Gathering held at a retreat center in the Catskills of New York in 1989. We sat next to each other before a pipe ceremony began and had a chance to chat.[11] I found out later that she was the matriarchal head of the Seneca Wolf Clan and lived on the Cattaraugus Reservation outside Buffalo, New York. Through a friend at the time I heard about the Women's Council she was hosting in June of the following year. I wanted to go and in fact I did attend.

At the Seventh Women's Council, held at the reservation in 1990, Grandmother shared the following story with us at this gathering. It concerned her mother's sense and need to find a way to pass down their clan's teachings. Also, she knew these teachings would be shared with the dominant culture.

She told us this story: Twylah's mother felt it really important to discuss the clan's teachings at length. The wolf is the tribal historian. The Wolf Clan then is responsible for keeping the history of the Seneca Nation intact. What vehicle could they use to interpret these teachings traditionally passed down in an oral way? Typewriters were being replaced by

17

computers. Libraries were in every community. The dominant culture did not learn through the oral tradition. Inspired, these women realized that the clock face could be used to impart these teachings using the circle and the numbers within the clock face to represent the wheel. The clock has twelve numbers with the thirteenth represented by the center of the clock. They also knew from their prophecies that the "flower" children of the 1960's and others would seek out Native elders, thirsty for knowledge and for a deeper understanding of human connection to this earth, something more than just working in factories, tearing up land for endless building. And it was happening. Folks from all walks of life began to seek out Native elders for their wisdom and traditions.

These two women had the opportunity to share something of a philosophy, a way of life, a respect for this earth, her resources that could shape our relationship with earth and nature and more. Their nation's teachings would be explained and recorded using this format. The circle, like a clock, gave a starting point for disseminating these teachings. The face of a clock offers twelve places with the center representing thirteen – a circle where lines and lessons could be placed, though it appears linear. These women knew it was a sphere of learning that was multidimensional. A circle has no beginning and no end. This reflects the totality of space, the universe, an understanding of the world that is the foundation of their Native American beliefs and many other cultures.

Meeting Grandmother Twylah, hearing her stories, the philosophy behind the wheel (her mother had passed away by this time), and after reading and learning about the four directions and elements from other Native American elders, I began to understand some of the concepts behind the Medicine Wheel. This circle that marks the four directions, that holds teachings, became a symbolic and metaphorical model for my life.

This model of understanding for life anchored me in the meadow. It became a part of me, a reference point for daily life.

Although I was not raised in a Native American community, I have that lineage. During that time, I sat in many circles with herbalists who had Native American teachers and with Native elders. We would anoint ourselves and the room with burnt sage for cleansing and preparation. Prayers, singing, drum beats opened the conversations and I learned their lore.

In these moments, I absorbed these teachings as if thirsty for the meaning and truths they represented. I watched and observed, listened, so that the wheel became a structure and a form for guiding the everyday. It felt right.

I attended the Seventh and Tenth Women's Councils in 1990 and 1993. Unfortunately they are no longer held. Here I learned about the Seneca "Cycles of Truth" as taught by Grandmother Twylah.

Each number on the wheel represents a truth. For example, number one, represents January, the color orange, and where "we learn the truth". Each tribe has a color for each direction and each direction holds the energy of the teaching. For example, the Seneca Nation has their system, which is different from the Lakota Nation.

I saw the Seneca wheel's "Cycles of Truth" come alive when I went to the Woman's Councils. Grandmother shared with us at the Women's Council her dream of a lodge, a physical place to share her teachings.

In the back of her home on the reservation, Grandmother's husband built this lodge for her. He based the design on her dream, constructing a circular structure with four doors and eight windows, two windows placed between each door so that the windows and doors equaled twelve.

Each door was placed and opened in one of the four cardinal directions – East, South, West, and North. The windows were the places in between. There in the center, Grandmother placed an altar and fire pit. The lodge was around twenty to forty feet in diameter, a large space, and when we walked inside to take a seat, we were encouraged to pay attention to where we sat.

Two cement steps were created around the entire inner periphery and were symbolically painted; the colors used inside were specific to the Seneca clan. The first steps were painted in the color of that direction. Therefore one quarter of the circle was painted in that specific color. For example, black was painted in the west quarter. The second step was painted in the colors of the twelve places on the wheel. All had meaning. As I mentioned previously, the first place on the wheel was painted orange.

Therefore, when we sat down, we were asked to consider, what direction were we in? What position on the wheel were we in? What was occurring in our life in that moment or in general where the teachings could speak to us? What learning was getting our attention?

At the first Women's Council that I attended in 1990, eighty plus women participated. We set up tents outside the lodge where an array of tents, from pup to the fanciest Coleman model, dotted the lawn. As we helped each other set up, we chattered like a convention of geese before winter's journey. In the way of women, it seems always and everywhere that we had stuff to unpack and set up. I chuckled as I looked around that first day and thought how we arrived in "horse" powered engines. That day, I felt I was coming home to something.

At the Tenth Women's Council held in 1993, Grandmother Twylah introduced us to Maka Nupa, a Cherokee and Lakota elder. Several years later she and I had a chance to meet, to sit together and get to know one another, become friends. As a teacher of this knowledge, she shared many stories and the wisdom of using this wheel of learning with me and others. She shared solutions to problems discovered as she used this system. While naturally intuitive, this wheel became a tool she readily shared and one I enjoyed learning about. She encouraged me to use the wheel as a tool for my own growth and development. What was my unique perspective and the wisdom I discovered, she asked? Then apply what I learned into my daily life.

Around the same time I began to study Native American teachings, I also came across the Sanskrit mandala as an art form.[12]

The Eastern traditions of Asia teach that the circle, the mandala, takes the formless and brings it into form and that the whole universe can be held and represented in this form. I became interested in meditation and the art form of the mandala. I began to draw from my meditation experiences and what I saw in dreams. This practice of placing dream images within a mandala or circle revealed much to me.

As the mandala can reveal our deepest self, the unconscious self, these drawings became another tool in the exploration of self and my relationship to the outer world. What could I uncover and reveal to myself that I was blind to?

This was and is no easy task, this facing of self, but I was hooked. My thirst for learning here in Eastern tradition and in the experiences of my Native American elders expanded and overrode any internal trepidations: What would I have to face again, what needed to be healed, how could I expand into more? The understanding of the four directions in any system takes patience and time to gain insight and wisdom.

A vital part of these teachings is to live them. Workshops bring knowledge but do not bring change. Rather, it is the practical application of these teachings that deepens our self-knowing, that enriches the everyday. Over time, I applied these principles in my everyday life.

Plants came in by nature's design not mine. I grew inside as I applied the teachings of the Medicine Wheel as I understood them. I crafted outside spaces into pathways in the form of symbols over about three to five years. When life pressed in on me, I would go into my backyard meadow either walking the spiral path or the Medicine Wheel. I became conscious of the four directions, the four elements, the thirteen places and teachings. I walked carefully in my desire to honor all species.

Whether outdoors or indoors, depending on the season and the weather I began and continue to begin my day with prayers and devotions to the four directions. I use sage when possible, tobacco if I have it and am able to release this small pinch to the earth, and I begin.

I want to give you a sense of the richness of each direction and a glimpse into its depths. The following section will present you with a brief review of some of the highlights I have come to appreciate over the years. I invite you to begin a wheel on paper marking the four directions and filling in some of these teachings, adding your own.

THE EAST

The East represents the dawn, springtime, infancy and childhood, yellow, air, illumination, clarity. Every morning's ritual began in the East, facing that direction. I knew the arc of the sun at morning's first light and how the sun travels and the arc shortens as winter drew near. Soon a bright yellow disc rises up over the horizon and brings light and warmth to our life.

It is said the darkest hours are just before the dawn when night shadows press in for whatever the mind cannot let go of. I know that to be true. One cannot walk the wheel of life without tasting something of its flavors or knowing emotions that prey on our minds and hearts. Dawn is welcomed after such nights of soul searching – problem tossing isn't it? The light comes in and chases away the monsters that try to keep a grip on our psyche. This knowing in morning's light washes away residues of night visions, soothes troubling dreams, and ignites the day.

Looking to the East then, is part of every morning's ritual. When I sit in the East with a concern, I ask for enlightenment and illumination. I try to see the concern with fresh eyes, even through the eyes of a child. Young children rub the sleep from their eyes. I cherished my children's giggles and boundless energy as our day began. Bright-eyed, open to wonder, curiosity for the new day are refreshing qualities to remember.

One of the most common symbols of the East, shared by many tribes and many cultures, is the eagle. The eagle flies the highest of the birds and is said to take our prayers to the Creator and to return with the answers.[13]

The eagle's view is expansive. When I see images of earth from outer space, I feel awe and envy the eagle: blue skies and swirling clouds, oceans and lands seem connected. Worries and fears wash away with the awareness of something more. But my vision can be limited. The eagle inspires me to look beyond the obvious, put my vision on an expanded view, to ride the currents of trust for a bit. Lift myself up from the mundane.

The East then, is the place of new beginnings. It is the place I begin the day. I face the East as I begin my morning's ritual. East speaks to the dawn and the start of a new day, of spring, of infancy, of eagle and air, of sunlit yellow and of the delicious moisture in dew or freshness of a lace of frost in winter. It is the time of the newborn baby, of the young fawn born in spring, of the first steps of a child.

When the dew begins to disappear as the sun rises, when frost leaves, the wheel moves towards noon. Noon represents the South, the second direction of prayer and acknowledgement.

THE SOUTH

The South represents noon, summer, adolescence, red, and the coyote. The South to me is bright and bouncing, like a teenager eager to grow, to shout, to play, to fill out its unique blossom and form, to reach and expand. This growing time, the summer, brings us flowers and seeds, vegetables and fruits, the medicines and nourishment we hope for if we plant and prepare correctly. Some develop right away; some take longer, but either way our gardens fill in and fill up with color and scent. The meadow does too. Bugs come, weeds compete: how does our garden grow? The same with adolescents. They come into their height, find their voice, fill-up and out with their unique expressions.

Late spring and through the summer, mid to late morning is a good gathering time. The morning wetness is gone, though I admit to going out early to walk on moist grass and see the sunlight sparkle in dew, casting thousands of small rainbows. Mid to late morning gathering of plants captures the plants' rising energy and freshness before the noon sun beats down. In the summer, when noon approaches and the hot sun gets higher in the sky, plants shut down a bit to conserve water.

Whether in our meadow or backyard or in our hearts, the South brings great activity. From buzzing bees to stinging wasps, beneficials and pests, each has its purpose and its consequences. With organic soil and companion planting in our gardens and diversity in the meadow, we see the benefit of the South. The South gets us into the dirt, pulling weeds, sculpting, shaping, and tending new growth as the season of summer touches through each day. In human terms, the energy of teenage years pops like the explosion of colors, tastes, and smells of a farmers' market. Music blares, days are later, tremendous growth emerges, both external and internal. Some days are hot and humid and seem to last forever. Then, thunder and lightning break summer's heat wave, bringing rain as teenage tensions break with new understandings.

Many Native American tribes connect the coyote with the direction of the South. Coyote is known as the trickster. He reminds us to lighten up, not take each other too seriously, sorely needed when the intensity of adolescent emotions sparks or when predatory pests invade the garden. Coyote reminds us too that the teenager will pull our chains, test our mettle, run over our feelings in their search of self. Can we handle the heat, put up sturdy fences of purpose, and stay true to our ideals when the going heats up? Can we laugh, giggle, and run through the hose on a hot summer day, dance and be light hearted and remember we really were once teenagers too?

When I lived in New England, summer found me sitting in the meadow and listening to the bees hum, intent on gathering nectar provided by the meadow plants. I appreciated the sun's light and heat, for in New England some summers were cloudy and the season short. There at the edge of the woods, I delighted when I caught sight of coyote's bushy tail at the forest line.

Red, fire, coyote, summer, adolescence, early adulthood, flowers coming and going, action and consequences, digging in dirt, all represent the South. Carl Jung, whose work in psychology and cognitive development focused on archetypes, felt that the South designated the shadow time when we have access to an interior pool of dark thoughts, emotions, and fears – those images that are in the shadows of our minds.[14]

When I sit in the South, I remember the shadow side of my nature. What is it I prefer to be hidden? What shadows are revealed in nighttime dreams, what aspects can I choose to face to help me understand myself? Gardens prepare us to accept the dirt and the mud, to stir the compost of rotten food, decaying grasses, manure, and sand to prepare the soil for new growth and new emergence.

As the sun moves closer to the Western horizon evening comes. Twilight, a time of supper and resting after the day's activities, brings stillness. The wind quiets down. In New England, I lived on top of a hill where the wind blew most days, bringing the constant sound of leaves gently rustling. This steady tempo quieted with the evening, when evening brings us to the West on the wheel.

THE WEST

The West for me is autumn, the adult years, the harvest, a time of reflection, introspection. Did I accomplish what I set out to do, those plans made with the morning's excitement? What's left as the day comes to a close? How's the drying going? Is any plant ready to be put into jars for storage? In the summer, I would often sit outside in late afternoon, waiting for twilight when fireflies would begin an exuberant dance at the tree line and bats would commence their aerial hunt. At dusk, peepers would sing and a few chirps could be heard from the birds settling in for the night. As I waited, I would sit at the base of one of my favorite trees, feeling the rough bark at my back and the grasses underneath in this stillness.

West is the twilight of the day's cycle, the time of the mature adult – one who has experienced the ups and downs of life, and of autumn, the bear, water, and blue. Here we understand that actions have consequences. If our humor has not disappeared with life's trials and tribulations, we understand more fully that life is transient and that nothing lasts forever. We have suffered losses and gains. West can be a time to forge ahead to new places, to move on, packing our bags into a new dream. We pull in; clean up the gardens, stock the woodpile for winter's quieter time.

Native American tribes often connect the bear to the West. The cave of the bear's hibernating time represents the dream time; the cave of the bear and its hibernation pattern is a symbol for the dark waters of our unconscious or subconscious mind, those aspects often revealed in dreams. Bear is the herbalist, the forager of the forest locating honey, berries, and other foods. Bears fear nothing and are strong, playful, the dreamer. They are practical and prepare for winter in the fall by getting fatter to sustain them through winter's sleep.

When we watch nature and observe the patterns of animals, we begin to awaken to the complexity of life. Like the bear, in late summer and early fall depending on the crop, we gather food for winter's use. Humans can, freeze, and dry food for storage. Canned peaches popped open on a cold winter's day remind us of the garden's sweetness. Hearty soups and stews filled with nourishing veggies warm us. A pot of tea, filled with summer flowers and leaves, joins friends and family around our table, fostering community.

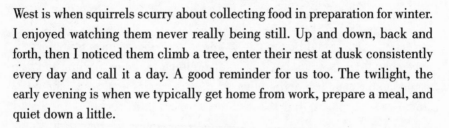

West is when squirrels scurry about collecting food in preparation for winter. I enjoyed watching them never really being still. Up and down, back and forth, then I noticed them climb a tree, enter their nest at dusk consistently every day and call it a day. A good reminder for us too. The twilight, the early evening is when we typically get home from work, prepare a meal, and quiet down a little.

The West is the place of the water element. Water from an archetypal framework is often connected to emotions.[15] Archetypes are defined as patterns, derived from the experience of the race and present in the unconscious of the individual. Dreams carry our deep emotions and unconscious thought to the surface for review and revelation. Dreams give us the opportunity to delve into the still waters of our psyche.

They can be especially helpful once we understand that dreams are given to us in symbolic language. Spending time to understand my dream symbols was invaluable and helped me to "crack the code", so to speak, of my dream symbols. What did specific dream symbols mean to me?

Dreams give us the opportunity to delve into the still waters of our psyche. I enjoyed bear's reminders of the importance of dreams. I kept journals. I would and still review them in morning's light. What nuggets are coming to the surface of my consciousness? What messages are relevant for the day?

Water, like each element represented on this wheel, is vital to life. My elders taught me to give thanks for the water we drink, cook with, bathe and play in. Water has been abused in our lifetime, polluted, tainted so much so we now buy it and hope it's really purified as advertising wants us believe.

The aqua blue of Caribbean waters, the deep turquoise and royal blues of the Pacific Ocean, the greens and browns of river water claim us and encourage us in some way to pay attention, breathe, and give thanks. Even the bear derives great joy and sustenance from fishing in the water.

When night is fully present and we settle down and go to sleep, the midnight hours roll in. The wheel moves towards the North. Midnight represents the North, winter, wisdom.

THE NORTH

When the day finishes, we enter the night, dark and mysterious, a time to replenish and rest. This is the place of our elders, our ancestors, winter, storytelling, buffalo, white or purple, earth, a time of thanks. The North is the dark of the night where we are guided by the light of the moon and her cycles. The elders know this planet is guided by a specific rhythm of cycles. There is a time to be born, a time to grow and live, a time to die, only to be born again. We live by the cycle of day and night, the four weeks of a moon waxing and waning, the cycle of seasons as the earth rotates around the sun.

I see these truths and these patterns in other models, not just those of Native Americans. This theme is repeated in Eastern traditions, in Aboriginal traditions on other continents.

When we are in the elder of our life we have the opportunity to share, to help from the experienced wisdom we carry as we have walked through dark and light. What can we share? How can we be available to our community? In the North we can see the lessons of the South differently. We are no longer teenagers intent on saving the world. We know we can save the world by being true to self and living an integrous life. If we truly want peace in our world, we have to be at peace in our daily life. We know change does not happen overnight. We can bring our levity and our humor to the younger ones for we know the pitfalls and the ecstasies are worth the climb.

We need our elders. Caroline Myss, author, teacher of spirituality and mysticism, suggests we have placed our old ones in the category of elderly instead of elders and that we no longer value their place in the community.[16]Are we afraid of growing old? If so, why? Can we not see a grace in our elder years, appreciate the seeds that bloomed, the fruit we tasted? What stories can we tell that breathe life and vibrancy to a life well lived, a life that learns and develops the muscle to go forth and maybe to reach upward for the sky?

When I heard Grandmother Twylah's introduction at the Seventh Women's Council, I was struck by the fact that she was described as the sum of all her experiences. How often do we appreciate ourselves and our elders in this way? Other elders I met along the way enjoy telling their stories and being asked to do so is a gift in itself. As listeners, what is the moral, the nugget in that story? Often when I asked a question or expressed puzzlement over an issue, the elder I sat with would tell a story, often personal. It was up to me to get it. They would not tell me what to do but gave me the space to hear in the story what I could understand in that moment. In one of my holistic health classes, Cross Cultural Health and Healing, I have the students read a story aloud as a class and then we discuss what they heard in that telling. Everyone hears something, and I had no doubt it was perfect for them.

The North brings us to the elders, our ancestors, and to storytelling and thanksgiving, white, quiet, midnight, prayer, and the spirit of white buffalo. The buffalo is earthy, massive, a roamer of the plains, and gives away so we humans have food, clothing, and tools. The white buffalo is thought to signal a time of abundance. The hump of the buffalo can represent a store of reserves. Athletes, for example, reach into a place of letting go and push forth from unknown reserves to win the title, the race. A mother or a father working two jobs has to find the reserves to provide for their family. Today with the economics of higher fuel prices and reduced house values we have had to dig into our creative reserves to find solutions to pressing personal or societal problems. The North reminds me to be humble, to know I cannot do it alone. What gifts have I accumulated as I look around the wheel? What am I grateful for today?

There is a wisdom and a humbleness here in honoring all our relations, the gifts of the harvest, the memory of spring's warmth, summer's blossom, and autumn's harvest.

New England snow and cold kept me inside, reading, playing games, visiting, poring over garden catalogs, and dreaming. The flow of seasons is to be cherished as nature's reminder to follow the seasons, not just in an outer way but to follow the tempo and gifts of each more deeply in our dreams and plans.

Spring passes and one remembers one's innocence.
Summer passes and one remembers one's exuberance.
Autumn passes and one remembers one's reverence.
Winter passes and one remembers one's perseverance.

—Yoko Ono, Japanese-American artist and musician

Flowers: The Medicine Wheel of Plants

The four seasons, the four directions, and the cycles of the year are all part of the Native American Wheel and other cultures; its teachings are complex, deep, inspiring, a compass. I shared with you the teachings I gathered in from the Seneca Nation, Grandmother Twylah Nitsch in particular and others. I also shared, to some degree, the way I assimilated them in my daily life and especially in my dreams. In the writing of this book I realized how many years this wheel has been a part of my consciousness. I understand that the application of a truth in our daily life is where the gifts lie.

I would like to relate a story from the Tenth Women's Council held in 1993, at the Cattaraugus Reservation in Buffalo, New York at Grandmother Twylah's home and lodge. It is a story that prodded me to think about taking the plants I was learning and placing them on a mandala wheel following the Cycles of Truth. However, before we convened for this women's event in June, a hurricane devastated Miami earlier in the year.

Three women from Miami stood before us and told us how difficult it was to get food and water into neighborhoods. Streets were filled with debris. Supply trucks could not get through. Folks had to band together to help each other out. But when food and water supplies are cut off what can we do in the moment? Their message to us, especially those of us who were working with the plant nations was: really get to know them, understand what parts are edible, how to use them medicinally. Gathering this knowledge can contribute to community. No one can take knowledge away from us.

When I returned home that June weekend, I sat in the meadow wanting to create my own plant wheel based on the Cycles of Truth, the teachings that Grandmother Twylah and others had shared at these councils. I said prayers, set my intention, and gave thanks. I quieted my mind and sat in the stillness stating I wanted guidance about my work with the plants nations and my intention to place them on a wheel for learning and guidance. I felt this was a way for me to learn about thirteen plants and use them in practical ways. And if I incorporated Grandmother Twylah's Cycle of Truth what would be revealed? How would this exercise foster my knowledge of the plants?

I sat this day in my meadow with sage and tobacco, set my intention, and asked, "How do I begin placing plants on a wheel for learning?"

In a while I heard: *"We'll help strengthen the connection."*

I persisted. "I really need to know the Devas, recognize them as separate from me, to hear them. Will you help?"

"We'll help. Persist. All answers are yours."

"Where do I begin? Who should I start with first?"

"Several."

But that confused me. I continued to write in my journal the stream of thoughts I heard.

"List us (the plants) here as you know them."

I made the following list of some of the common plants in my meadow:

Plantain, *Plantago major*

Nettles, *Urtica dioca*

Yarrow, *Achillea millefolium*

Coltsfoot, *Tussilago farfara*

Self-Heal, *Prunella vulgaris*

Wild Strawberry, *Fragaria vesca*

Rose, *Rosaceae*

Goldenrod, *Solidago canadensis*

Poison Ivy, *Rhus toxicodendron*

Dandelion, *Taraxacum officinalis*

Mullein, *Verbascum thapus*

Purple Coneflower, *Echinacea spc*

Meadow flowers (this is a general name)

This was my list for the thirteen places on the wheel. I continued to sit quietly.

"Now, place us as you named us on your Cycles of Truth wheel and see what happens."

My uncertainty still showed up with this kind of inspiration. Was it real? Was this just my wishful thinking?

"How do I begin with you?" I asked again.

"Sit and listen. Start with us one at a time. Bring each plant into your meditation. That is how you begin connecting with us. Write all thoughts and then move to the next plant. Allow the flow. Record all impressions. Start with what you've learned. Allow us to work with you."

I did. It took a while, but the following plant wheel is the result of the above guided efforts. Observing, listening became invaluable skills to hone. Intuitive knowing takes practice and diligence to refine. During this process I opened a gate into a realm of understanding, one different from the path of the scientifically trained mind. I also found that placing twelve plants on this wheel gave me a reference point of learning.

1. Learning the Truth: Plantain (Plantago major)

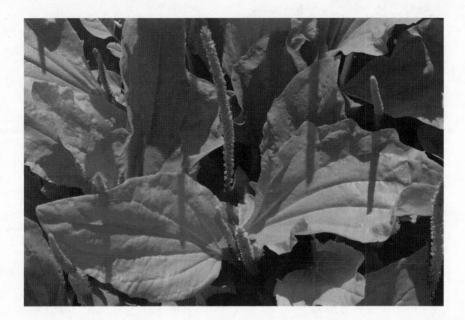

What does learning the truth mean to you? I am a seeker, a lover of learning. There are times I have devoured books with the ease of eating a bag of M&M's. For me it is the place of beginning a project, an undertaking, a new subject. I feel the excitement and the freshness of the new discoveries here. I can't wait to finish the book, the concept and take it to my within. Learning the truth has joy and pain. Both sides are a part of life.

Pam Montgomery, my first herbal teacher, introduced me to plantain.[17] Pam, slender, hair streaked with silver, lived at that time on an orchard where part of the orchard overlooked the Hudson River in upstate New York. She was beginning her journey as an herb teacher. She helped manage the vegetable growing for the owner's family farm stand.

We walked up and down fields on a beautiful, sunny afternoon as she pointed out edible and medicinal plants. She taught me how to gather, wash, cut, and pack plantain in a jar. She added olive oil and together we made my first infusion. With some oil already infused, we made a salve. Plant material was strained. We added a specific amount of beeswax to the quantity of oil used in order to create a salve of desired consistency. Beeswax helps solidify the oil.

While we worked, she continued to highlight the benefits of this plant. When stung by a bee or bitten by mosquitoes, she taught me that one can chew fresh leaves which puts saliva in the mix. This mash can then be applied to a bee sting or bite. A salve made from the whole plant can be used for all manner of scrapes, abrasions, bruises. She suggested that this one plant, made into an oil and a salve, can be the beginning of a home medicine chest.

Plantain became my first connection to the medicinal plant world. This little "weed" is often the first plant that beginner herbalists learn about. I say "weed" because anyone who wants a golf-course-smooth lawn grows to dislike this tenacious grass filler. But not herbalists. This plant is known as the "band aid" plant.

Like its name implies, it can be used for many minor cuts, blisters, bites, and scrapes. It tends to grow by the garden's disturbed soil edges. If one walks across a lawn and compacts the grass, plantain will show up.

Little did I know as I began my journey that my trained scientific mind would have to step aside as I started to observe. I delved into the herb books and soaked up what learning I could, but observation and patience are the real teachers in the plant world.

Time and patience to watch and work with a meadow through all seasons became part of my training. Season after season I gained a new respect for nature. I watched where on the horizon the sun rose and set; where did the moon rise? I listened to the wind for we lived up on a hill and sometimes the wind rolled boisterously through the surrounding hills. It is the soft breezes playing at the forest border in the afternoon that I remember the most.

After my visit with Pam, I was fired up. I went home and rushed out to our backyard. I looked at the "grass" in the back third of the property and did not see grass. Later I invited Pam out and she identified several medicinal plants. I decided I would like to let the back third grow and see what showed up. I eagerly waited to see what spring and summer brought in. In the meantime, plantain was as easily found as mentioned above. I gathered it and began to make my first infusions. Infusion means I gathered plants, washed and cut, filled a mason jar about two-thirds full and then filled with a liquid, or menstruum. In this case I used extra-virgin olive oil. This is known as an infusion. I placed the jar in a sunny location and let sit for six weeks. This one plant became a handy remedy for a variety of situations.

These are some of the stories I share with my students.

One day my sons, probably ages five and eight, were playing with cousins in the woods that bordered the back of our property. Wielding sticks, they traipsed over the colonial stone wall and poked their sticks right into a yellow jackets' nest. Angry wasps went on the attack. Amid screeches and screams, two boys came flying into the yard vigorously swatting these tiny armed flyers. I gathered everyone and pointed out plantain plant and got everyone to pick a leaf and start chewing. Chewing the leaf breaks open the cell wall and releases the healing properties.

Please keep in mind my yard was organic. We did not use pesticides or lawn fertilizers. We placed chewed leaves on every bite, and both boys had at least fifteen to twenty of them on head, neck, and arms.

The more severe bites were covered with a bit of plant material and then a band-aid was put on them to keep the plant in contact with the skin bite. The boys were checked before bedtime. Many of the bites were not red. A few appeared more severe. To these we put on a new application of chewed plant material and a band aid. Neither boy complained of itching. In the morning, they seemed fine. There were still one or two red areas so we reapplied new plant material. There was no swelling or signs of an allergic reaction in either boy.

I tried the same method on myself with a bee sting. I had been gathering red clover, and bumblebees like to hang out upside-down underneath the flower. I did not see the bee and got stung. I picked a plantain leaf, chewed it, and applied it to the sting. Within 20 minutes or so, the stinging stopped. I applied new plant material and a band-aid that night. I too never awakened with a maddening itch that I remembered from bites and stings I had got going barefoot as a child.

Another incident occurred later that gave me another opportunity to learn something different about plantain. One evening I was out walking with my neighbors. The developer had created a circle of homes that made a good walking track. My neighbors and I walked for about two miles chattering away about kids and school. When I returned home I found myself with blisters about two by three inches on the bottoms of my heels. I knew when blisters broke and the tender dermis under the skin was exposed it could be painful. I had a family to take care of and I became concerned that if the skin tore and oozed it would interfere with my day. I got out my herb books and discovered that the Native Americans used plantain leaves to help with blisters. The recommendation was to soak fresh leaves in vinegar and leave out overnight, then place on blisters in the morning. I did just that. As a precaution I gently rubbed some of the oil I was infusing on my heels before I went to bed. In the morning I placed the wilted leaves soaked in vinegar between sock and foot and then began my day.

The day rolled by and I really did not give my feet any thought. By late afternoon I decided to check my heels. I removed my socks easily, as nothing was sticking. I found that the water had drained from the blisters without any bleeding or irritation and that the skin had stayed in place. I was amazed and delighted that I had been walking without discomfort. Soon the blistered skin healed. Yes, I applied the oil again at night probably for two or three nights. And yes, the second day I placed the vinegar soaked leaves between sock and foot before donning shoes. It worked.

Plantain works well on healing scrapes and abrasions. Again, while studying this plant, another incident occurred that gave me an opportunity to use plantain. My younger son, about five or six years old, fell off his bike by the side of the road where there was a lot of gravel. With tears streaming down his cheeks I saw abrasions from forehead to chin including his upper lip. We went into the house and washed all the cuts and then applied the plantain salve. He accepted the salve on forehead and chin, but refused to have me put some on his upper lip. A week went by. The abrasions on forehead and chin healed without any signs of infection or scarring. However, he noticed the abrasions on his upper lip were not healing as fast and some still remained. He asked me to put the salve on them and we did, twice a day. Placing some before school and at night did the trick. All his abrasions healed with no scarring.

My sons played soccer most of their school years. Both came home after many a game with slide tackle burns and abrasions from the hip to mid-thigh. We would clean them off and then apply plantain salve. If these abrasions were particularly raw, we would cover them overnight with sterile gauze, repeating this at night until the danger of reopening was past. Usually in a day or two gauze was no longer needed. Skin healed and we never had any infections.

I have made this salve dozens of times. I usually include three other herbs that are known for wound healing. I often give a sample to my university students to take home and try. One student shared this story: Her mother had been bothered by a severe skin irritation on her feet. Nothing relieved the intense itching. She had been to doctors and tried all sorts of creams, etc. She applied the plantain salve I handed out to the students that night. Her daughter came into class the next day and reported that her mother slept the whole night and did not wake up itching. She was surprised and relieved that something helped.

During this time my aunt had rental property on Cape Cod. She would often have cracked skin from the frequent use of cleaning products. She would rub the salve on her hands and then wear cotton gloves for the night. She woke up with relief. Her cracked skin healed quickly using the salve in this way.

A customer of mine was/is still a glass blower. If one drop of molten glass drops onto her skin it's an immediate third-degree burn. She would buy the salve to keep in her studio. She observed that the burn would be fifty percent healed overnight with one application of this salve.

In medicine these stories are considered testimonials. Hardly scientific, they relate the practical uses of this plant in practical everyday ways. I saw many geriatric patients with bedsores and often wondered if these simple salves could work. In the folkloric tradition, these uses are valid. It is how medicine was passed down through the ages. We forget that a lot of trial and error went into the use of plant medicines. The remedies that work are still with us today.

We have forgotten also how nature provides for us. My Native American friends would often remind me that there is a remedy for every ailment if we but pay attention. I have and continue to use plantain as my remedy of choice for bites, cuts, scrapes, and blisters. I always scout out the area where I live and often find these plants. I give talks and plant walks on wild edibles, and plantain is often the first plant I talk about. While my children were growing up, I stopped using, nor did I have need for, antibiotic or steroid ointments. Plantain and other plants have antibiotic-like, antiseptic properties. Trained in Western medicine, I had to learn to harvest each plant at its appropriate time and learn to use it properly. I evaluated the results myself and listened to students and friends as they used it to heal skin issues. If healing does not occur easily or an infection should arise then there are other plants that can be called in.

I learned many facets of herbalism in my beginning steps. Here's a beginner's list:

1. Use three to five reliable plant guides to identify a plant. Check it out with someone who knows the plants.

2. Never taste a plant in the wild you do not know.

3. Common names can be two different species, and it's possible one could be poisonous. Learn the botanical names whenever possible. For example, when I mention plantain on herb walks, many folks automatically assume the banana plantains, which are in the Musa genus, not Plantago, and are tropical.

4. I learned how to make a tea, decoction (a medicinal form of tea), tinctures, and salves.

5. Learning what parts of the plant to use happened slowly as I discovered each plant.

6. Learning when was the best time to harvest each plant also happened as I studied each one.

These observations are useful and contributed to my learning, the beginning steps I took into the world of herbalism.

2. HONOR THE TRUTH: NETTLES (URTICA DIOCA)

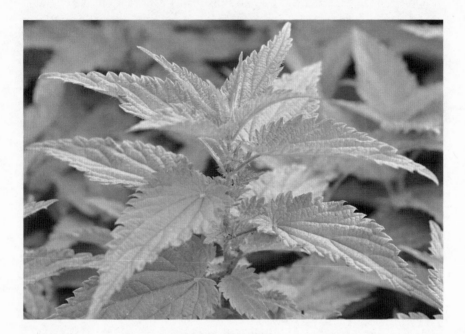

Honor has many implications. How do we honor ourself? Our community? The earth? In general, the word "honor" encompasses reputation, acting and respecting others. It is also a word that connotes giving or expressing to someone their due, valuing them in some way for their worth. "Honor the truth" holds the second place on this wheel.

Nettles, with square and downy stems, are covered with tiny, sharp spikes that release an acrid fluid when touched, much like a bee sting. Formic acid is released, and one is left with a pin dot mark, like a mosquito bite, that itches. This reputation to "sting" usually makes many wary. Some loathe to gather this plant, others consider it a nuisance.

Yet nettles are one of my favorite spring herbs. They are best gathered in early spring, usually when they are less than one foot tall. Later in the season they get gritty, accumulate crystals, cystolliths that make them unpalatable to eat. The leaves contain phosphorus and a trace of iron, chlorophyll, and vitamin C.

I gather for two reasons: one, to cook and eat that day; two, to dry for later use. Gathering requires me to become quiet before I stick my hand among the stalks. It is tricky to clip without getting stung. This plant gives us a challenge. I often remark to my students that nettles command respect. A calm and careful approach can reduce the stings when harvesting. Some herbalists like the stings and believe that the formic acid helps the joints. In fact, in the old herbals there are reports of those with arthritis using nettle stalks to slap against a joint, with the resulting stings stimulating circulation and providing relief from soreness or stiffness.[18]

Nettles are useful as a pot herb. This simply means boil water and throw some chopped up plant material in and let it sit in the "pot". Cooking neutralizes the sting and the cooked leaves are delicious. They can be eaten plain or added to any veggie dish.

Nettles, long valued as a tonic herb that strengthens the whole body, are also good for tea, something I enjoy in early spring. After gathering nettles, I chop the plants and spread on a cookie sheet to dry for tea making.

Nettle pesto, different from basil in flavor, is a treat. Again, fresh leaves are chopped and substituted in the traditional pesto recipe.

Nettle stems are valued for their fiber. While in herb school (in the mid-nineties I enrolled in Rosemary Gladstar's Herb Apprenticeship course), we separated the fibers using the cut and dried stalks gathered in late summer. We then wove our own cordage. Historically, this fiber was used in clothing, sailcloth, and sacking material.

Nettles are found in most temperate regions. They seemed to have followed the migration of man around the globe. Great in the compost pile, great feed for bovines, they have many uses and are valued by those who honor its worth.

3. KNOW THE TRUTH: YARROW (ACHILLEA MILLEFOLIUM)

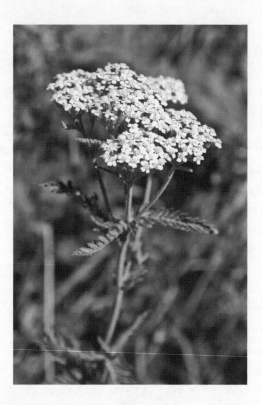

Knowing the truth can take life experience, years of study, or an intuitive hit that occurs in a split second. Every experience adds to the whole of us, giving us an understanding or an innate sense of what is best. Understanding the properties of a plant's makeup deepens our knowing of its uses. In knowing is knowledge, and knowledge strengthens our awareness and ability to harvest a plant at the appropriate time, use the appropriate plant part, and make the type of preparation that serves the needed purpose.

Soft and lacey, delicate leaves of yarrow hide among the grasses in early spring. This plant is one of the first I got to know as we let the "grass" grow in the first years of the meadow. I consider it one of the first to bring knowledge of a plant's medicine to me. By July, yarrow grows to about twelve inches or so, and then the white flowers bloom. They popped up here and there in the meadow, and that first season, I transplanted a few in my more formal garden. I noticed that when left on their own they seemed to move in a circular fashion from year to year. I first planted some on the east side, and the next spring I noticed they had moved counter-clockwise into the north side.

Yarrow has a perennial root structure and propagates itself from seeds formed in the spent flower heads. Tiny white flowers form and create flat heads. They bloom from July to September or longer depending on where you live.

When I watched the flowers appear, it became easy to tell when the flower waned.

This common meadow plant is not native to North America though it can be found in most places. It has many common names, which often give us a clue as to its colloquial and historic uses. The ancient herbals give reference to the use of yarrow as an aid to staunch blood from cuts and wounds. Yarrow helped wounds from inflictions in war times as well as served as a popular herb that carpenters used to stop bleeding. Because of these properties I put yarrow in my all-purpose salve.

A good example of its use occurred during one of the herbal apprenticeship classes I attended at Sage Mountain in Vermont. Rosemary Gladstar founded and ran herbal classes here. It is where I received my certificate in herbology after completing her comprehensive apprenticeship program.[19]

One of the cooks was carrying a large glass bowl with salad for our dinner. She tripped and fell down some stairs with the salad bowl in hand. She gashed her forearm and those nearest to her went in the nearby garden, picked some yarrow, and packed the gash. Plantain leaves were used as well. Off they went to the Emergency Room. The bleeding was staunched before they arrived, though she needed twenty-two stitches. The herb crew I am sure received some curious stares as this patient walked in with plant material stuck to her arm. But in the past, these plants were used to help a wound heal.

I tell this story because we have become afraid to use the common weeds around us first to help. Yes, it takes knowledge of the proper use. Once trained, I became less fearful and even marveled at what nature supplied beneath my feet. Pharmacy medicine has its roots in herbal medicine, and our meadows contain useful healing plants for many common ailments.

One of the basics in plant gathering for tincture or salve making is to know what plant parts are used and when to gather them. Yarrow flowers are best gathered just as they start to bloom. The leaves are also stripped from the stem. I cut flowers and leaves up into small pieces and fill a quart mason jar about two-thirds full and then add extra-virgin olive oil to the top. I place the lid on securely and then let it sit in a sunny windowsill, shaking the jar often. After five to six weeks, I strain the infused oil and use this oil in salve making. I keep some flowers and leaves aside to dry for teas and for my hiking backpack.

Yarrow also helps with colds. It has a peppery taste and combines well with other herbs and contributes a property that helps us sweat. Yarrow was commonly combined with other herbs to help move a cold through our system. A teaspoon with other herbs put in a pot is nourishing, and the vitamins and minerals, in trace amounts, contribute to overall health and well being. I met many a dedicated herbalist who radiates vibrant health and vitality who uses herbs for food and medicine in everyday life.

I was not a Master Gardener when I started and tended this meadow. I did not know the extent of the diversity of species I was attracting. But I can tell you I saw such variety of insects. Today I know that 4,500+ species are in peril. It takes variety in the landscape to support their life cycles. One pair of chickadees with three chicks eats 300 caterpillars per day.[20] As our landscapes shrink with urbanization, we are losing these populations.

Yarrow supports two important beneficials – ladybugs and hover flies, which eat aphids. Therefore it is a good companion plant for the garden. It can be a ground cover that helps with erosion control so planting on hillsides is a plus. There are many hybrids and variety of colors. *Achilles millefollium,* white yarrow, is what I used and continue to look for in the surrounding meadows where I live today, to replenish my supplies for tea or salve making.

Trying the herb in both tea form and salve contributes to my knowing how to use a plant and what effect it has. Through this practice, I gain applied knowledge and plant understanding.

4. See the Truth: Coltsfoot (Tusilago farfara)

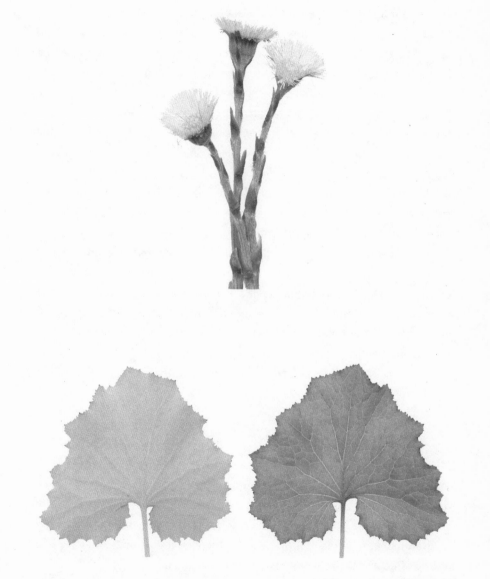

Seeing the truth involves more than the sense of sight. Feeling, intuitive knowing in our gut, sensing more than what is visible or relating what is visible in a different way can enhance our learning. Artists are great at that, are they not? Monet's impressions of pond and lilies still move us today. Michelangelo's *Pietà* and *David* are breathtaking masterpieces of seeing something within a formless slab of stone and making it manifest in the visible that fill us with the majesty of that inconceivable creation.

The Doctrine of Signatures was born from observations of the plant world and theology.[21] The reasoning of the ancients carried forth to this day is that God left his signature on all things more than we realize. They developed this idea in ancient times as a way of relating the form and shape of a plant to the form and shape of a body part or organ, and it is often referred to in herbal circles today. Thus the plant was said to help heal that body part that matched its shape. Knit bone, the common name of comfrey root, is said to help knit the bones. *Gingko biloba*, the most ancient tree on the planet, has lobed shaped leaves that resemble the lobes of the brain. Today extensive research is being conducted on the relationship of gingko's chemical constituents and healing of the brain.

In a class with David Winston, Cherokee Healer and Medicine Man, I learned that the color and shape of plants, smells, and forms can give us clues as to the possible functions of a plant or the way to name a plant to remember it for future use.[22] The yellowish root of dandelions suggests it can help with the balancing of the gall bladder/liver system, and in fact it does. Remember we do not eat yellow daffodils because they are toxic to the liver. The purple and blue flowers of skullcap are soothing to the nervous system.

My first experience with coltsfoot was accidental. As my children got a bit older, we decided to add an above-ground pool to our backyard. Dirt from the site selected was carefully removed and placed by the drip line of a grove of hemlocks. The dirt pile was spread evenly and not too high in order to allow moisture to reach the tree roots. Imagine my surprise the following spring when a semicircle of yellow, dandelion-like flowers appeared. At first I thought more dandelions were producing in the disturbed soil. When I looked closer I did not find any leaves. Curious, I went back to my herbal guides and discovered that coltsfoot flowers do in fact resemble dandelion flowers, but unlike dandelions, put up their flowers first. And unlike the smooth stem of a dandelion, coltsfoot shoots up a flowering stem with numerous reddish bracts and whitish hairs. When the flowers die off, leaves in the shape of a colt's foot appear. An old name for coltsfoot in the European herbals was *Filius ante patrem,* which means the son before the father.[23] That name captures the growing characteristic of this plant beautifully.

How is this plant used? The leaves are collected in early June, July at their freshest. Its common use is as a demulcent, expectorant, and tonic. Coltsfoot, for example, was and is used as a cough syrup.

Leaves and flower stems are placed in a quart of boiling water, and then the water slowly steams off leaving half the solution. I added honey to this tea and stored in the refrigerator to use when needed. I have come across other sources that suggest the flowers can be placed in a jar, adding raw honey and stored for a few weeks. This honey mixture is soothing for a dry cough or irritated throat. I found it effective in helping to stop a cough accompanied by a cold. My cough syrup keeps well in the refrigerator for about six to nine months, enough to get through a winter season.

In wilderness studies I learned that the leaves of coltsfoot can be burned almost to a crisp where they then can be crumbled or ground into a finer texture. When in this form, they can be added to a recipe as they contain potassium salts. This is a great tip for campers, hikers. Picking a few coltsfoot leaves is a good idea for when the day ends, the campfire gets going, and supper is cooking. The powdered leaves can be added as a seasoning. Plants rich in potassium help relieve edema, and help the body release fluids that can build up in the feet. Old herbals recommend inhaling the smoke for a persistent cough or even asthma. I have never tried this myself, though I would not be afraid to do so.

Young leaves and flowers of coltsfoot can be eaten although the leaves may taste better if first gently boiled before being added to salads or vegetable dishes.

Seeing the flower's growth pattern, observing the flower first, without leaves and then to see coltsfoot-shaped leaves is unforgettable. These plants are distinct and easy to spot by woodland trails, roadsides. Remember though,

I do not advise using plants by the roadside as they are contaminated with oils, tar, leads from cars, and road work.

This plant was a surprise received from disturbed soil, but soil that I knew was safe. What a gift and what a sight to behold!

5. Hear the Truth: Self-Heal, All Heal, Heal-All (Prunella vulgaris)

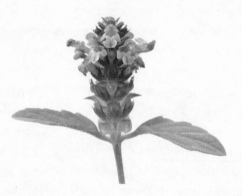

The definition of hearing and listening can be debated: Which one is more important? I have often heard folks say, "I know you heard me, but did you listen?" Listening then requires something more, doesn't it? Hearing what a person says and then listening for what's underneath is tricky. Yet hearing the truth requires the inner discipline to get one's self out of the way and focus on what and how something is being said. Listening to the wind has its own poetry. Some suggest there is a sound to the sunrise, to the forming of morning dew. Nature seems to vibrate on a different wavelength from human noise.

Plants have their own rhythm, trees dance with the wind, rocks crack against each other, waves crescendo towards the beach, clouds shuffle in endless patterns. Movement and sound are a part of nature, yet it seems we have forgotten how to hear nature except in casual passing or only when a storm barrels in. Again I am suggesting that when the crack and boom of a thunderstorm or of a river rushing into our basement gets our attention, we lose interest in the quieter sounds of what's around us. How would you describe the sound of a meadow growing? Can we describe the sound of our land moving through the seasons?

Our name carries a sound vibration much like the sound difference of a breeze or when the wind shifts with an incoming storm. The ancient ones taught that the vowels in our name are the vibration we enter this life on. What is your name? Do you like the sound of your name? Are you comfortable with the tone of your name? Does your name have special meaning to you, your family? If you are unhappy with your name, why? What is contained in the vibratory tone of speaking one's name that feels right or wrong?

I found the common names for *prunella vulgaris* intriguing. Self-heal, heal-all, and all-heal are a few of the common names for *prunella vulgaris*. Can a plant encompass healing self with a variety of ailments? Can one plant be so diverse, carry a broader talent? What is heard here in these names that implies this plant's purpose?

Self-heal is an example of how a common name can be descriptive of some of the properties of a common "weed". When I first spotted it in my meadow, I became curious as to its uses. I verified the plant using three to five field guides and asked for confirmation during herb gatherings. By this time I had seen several budding herbalists make salves, and they used more than one herb. I was pleasantly surprised to learn that self-heal is an excellent wound healer. In fact, the old herbals from the U.K. proclaim there is no better herb for wound healing. In doing research to make my own salve, I decided to add this one to the mix.

The whole herb is gathered in midsummer. This plant is popular with bees, who seek it out for its sweet nectar for honey making, but bees also assist in fertilization of these plants. I keep some dried in my medicine cabinet for use in the winter to ward off colds and flu. Recent research is proving the antiviral properties of this plant, and Chinese researchers are using this plant successfully to control gingivitis and herpes infections.[24]

Self-heal's reputation lies with its ability to help heal external wounds when it is applied as a poultice or salve. As an internal remedy, it can be added to a tea blend to relieve a cold. Add honey to tea made with self-heal and you have a pleasant remedy for sore throats.

I keep it for sore throats and general wellness when not feeling well. Many of the traditional herbalists extol its benefits to heal all inward and outward wounds and say that it is an excellent mouth rinse or gargle for mouth ulcers.

Self-heal can easily be confused with ground ivy, **Glechoma hederacea**. It's low-growing, found in lawns, and has a similar appearance. The little purple flowers at first glance seem to resemble **Prunella vulgaris**. Ground ivy comes a bit earlier, but look carefully at the plant structure of both to discern the difference.

Hearing the truth is contained in the name of this plant.

6. SPEAK THE TRUTH: WILD STRAWBERRY (FRAGARIA VESCA)

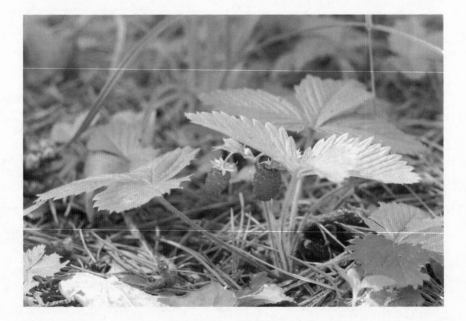

Speaking the truth for me involves the right use of words, intent behind the words, being mindful how I say the words. Am I communicating the truth?

How do I articulate my desires? How many times do I babble or rant to cover up my true feelings? Am I heard and do I allow others to speak? The Buddhists teach compassionate listening.[25] Can I allow another to speak before I have to jump in, tell my viewpoint? Speaking the truth has different facets that involve listening as well as speaking. I have often observed elders sitting and observing the folks in the group before speaking. Their assessments on the energies of the folks around often proved accurate.

Their culture and all I have read spoke to me of an understanding of nature. The four directions were spoken of in many ways, in many circles, as if to imprint upon us the value of knowing the elements that govern this planet, our home. Our media seems to reward the rants and raves of a few who spout distortions of the facts in endless monologues. To speak the truth in its highest form is a responsibility of the highest form. How many stories have you read of Native Americans who sat before the politicians of the day in silence? When they spoke it was to the point and then they were done.

Juicy, heart-shaped fruit of the wild strawberry can be found tucked under small leaves of its parent, mixed in with bedstraw and buttercup. I think it is a deliberate conspiracy between robins and crows, rabbits, and fairies to gobble them up before we get a chance to search for them in the meadow. Sweet and tasty, more flavorful than their cultivated cousins, wild strawberries can be found on the meadow's floor as part of its carpet. Low-growing, often mixed in with buttercups, they are found in between the stems and stalks of taller plants. I enjoy going out in the beginning days of summer to see how many delicious berries I can find.

Several Northeast Native American tribes name the moons after a common event, a marker for tribal life continuity. The Moon in June is often referred to as the Strawberry Moon, a reminder that the fruit ripens in June and for a couple of weeks can be picked, harvested, dried, and simply enjoyed as one of summer's delightful and precious treats. One of my Native American elder friends, Nupa Maka, rekindled the "Strawberry Moon Ceremony" that honors women. It is thought that the fruit is shaped like our wombs, and the red juice is likened to a women's menstrual flow. This plant became honored for many years with rites and rituals. The strawberry became a symbol of women's gifts, and the ceremony passed on women's teachings. The Strawberry Moon weekends I had/have the privilege of attending were/are filled with a sharing. Some of us stepped into the roles of teachers and we helped each other and offered support.

In herbalism, the color of the flower, the shape, the color of the root and juices can be clues as to some of the medicinal properties of a plant. These are the Doctrine of Signatures, observations as those mentioned earlier, which are being proven through Western scientific method to be true.

When I realized I had wild strawberry growing in my meadow I can tell you I was overjoyed. Fresh delicious strawberries were literally beneath my feet. I discovered that wild strawberry leaf as a tea and decoction offered relief from diarrhea, dysentery, gastric upsets, and intestinal weaknesses and was also a blood builder. Strawberry leaf tea is mild and pleasant.

I would often add small amounts of leaves, finely chopped, to my salads.

At herb gatherings, those women who specialized in women's herbs always included wild strawberry. Adele Dawson, in *Herbs, Partners for Life*, notes the safe use of this tea in pregnancy.[26] It can be used before and after delivery to help lactation since it is the mildest of the rose family. This author and herbalist also states: Strawberry leaf tea is "safe for infants who cannot tolerate other foods."

The Cherokee used strawberry leaf tea along with other plants as a refreshing and relaxing drink after long hunting trips.[27]

The strawberry speaks to me of the path of woman. She travels the path of maiden, mother (whether through her children or her creative gifts), and then hopefully to the time of the crone, the elder. Some mothers are good at setting examples for their daughters. We have forgotten though, the importance of our menstrual cycle, that we are the ones who bear children, who bring forth life, as my elders would say. I have counseled women with daughters and reminded them to take time with their daughters during their menses. Teach them to rest a bit, to let the creative juices stir, share stories, give a massage or go into nature together, and share dreams. It is said that our menses can be a powerful, creative and receptive time. To the women

I ask, how do you honor this time of the month? To the men I ask, please honor us again as your co-creative partners.

When we reach the end of our menstrual cycles we have the opportunity to share our stories with younger women from a place of experience. We take the truths we learned and can bring levity to situations, knowing nothing lasts forever and that life can change in a heartbeat. We have our sorrows and our joys, which fill us out and make our depths richer.

Little strawberry, hidden in the meadow's carpet, reminds me how important women's stories are. Storytelling is a gift of speaking the truth; for conveying lessons and morals. Good storytellers get our attention with raising a voice at a critical point, embellishing the tale with juicy tidbits, elaborating and exaggerating evil deeds or whispering that help is on the way. Ceremonies like the Strawberry Moon give all a voice, a chance to speak out and up. Tiny strawberry, vibrant red plays hide and seek, using its color and shape to speak its truth.

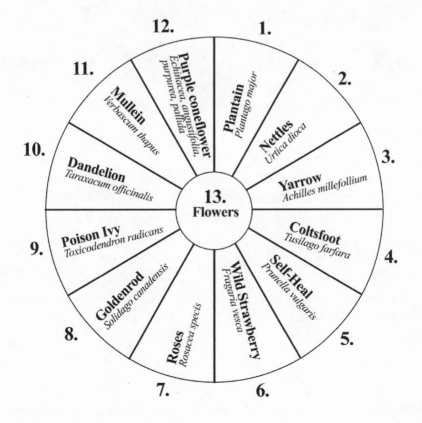

7. LOVE THE TRUTH:
ROSES (ROSACEAE AND SPS)

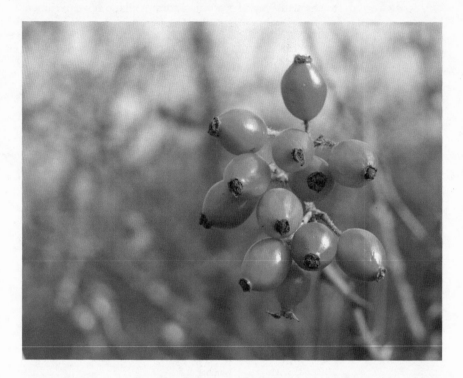

In delving into Medicine Wheel teachings, I came to understand that loving the truth is one of the hardest places on the wheel. We talk of romantic love, the love that brings a refreshing sweetness to our lives till the bloom fades. We talk of the love we feel for our babies, that unconditional feeling for the magic and mystery of creation we can hold in our arms. However, unconditional love is most needed in the places we find hard to love; places that are thorny, persistent, difficult to remove, entangled in a prickly mess and sometimes downright horrible. My teachers taught me that when we want love in our lives we often "get" to see the places where love is not. That is where loving the truth can be the hardest and most needed.

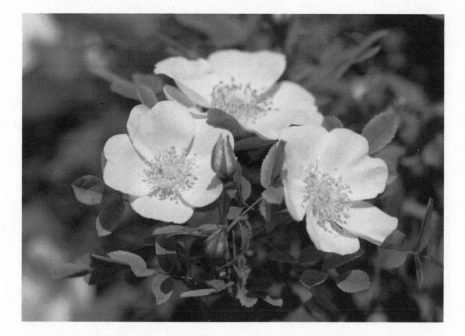

Poets and playwrights, gardeners and lovers know the rose to be a symbol of love's perfection. Soft petals open to the sun's light. Fragrant and lovely the rose is probably one of the most sought after plants and most revered. The number of hybrids clearly speaks to our love of the rose. How many colors can we create? Garden catalogs have pages and pages of old varieties and new. Sought after by kings and queens, the rose has undergone transformations in color, petals, and production. Rose of attar is highly prized fragrance, one that is expensive and used in perfumery, teas, and cooking.

It is said the rose heals the heart. Its fragrant smell can create a feeling of happiness. The rose has become a flower that enthralls most of us with her beauty, her scent in spite of her thorns. That is the paradox of unconditional love: to love another like ourself no matter the thorns.

I chose to follow the path of the wild rose. This dense, spreading shrub found along the wayside was introduced to the U.S. from Japan around the

1860's. It was originally cultivated as an ornamental for erosion control and as a living fence to prevent or deter livestock from wandering. However, the multiflora rose that is evident by our roadsides and forest edges is now considered an invasive. My yard in New England had wild roses in the forest edging. Some jumped into the heart of my meadow. I pruned vigorously a couple of times a year but chose not to rid the land of this species. The bushes left provided food and wildlife shelter and habitat.

I brought the flowers, soft white with pale pink coloring, into the house. Vases and baskets were placed in the main rooms and our bedroom. Often as twilight stole in, I would catch the fragrance on the evening breeze; it was heavenly. The wild rose blooms for about ten days in late May to early June, depending on New England's weather. If I did not stop to gather these lovely petals I would lament my loss till next spring's blooms.

One of my herbal teachers, Rosemary Gladstar, has a recipe for a soothing and creamy skin cream that I enjoyed making year after year.[28] I gather wild roses for beauty and to make this skin cream. I place wild rose petals in a quart mason jar, fill the jar with almond oil to the top, and let sit on a sunny windowsill. After about five to six weeks, I strain the oil, placing the petals in the compost pile.

For cooking, recipes abound using rose petals. Tea sandwiches, jams and jellies, puddings are examples of recipes easily found.

A word of caution: You must not use roses from florist shops as chemicals are used to treat them. Most of the imported roses to the U.S. come from Columbia and Ecuador, though European sources contribute. Our U.S. growers, predominately California and Florida, are finding it harder to compete with foreign sources. We import ninety percent of our roses from Columbia. Plant species are chemically treated to help them handle the handling, e.g., the length of trip, timed with optimal bloom time.

If you use rose petals, know your source and know that they are free of chemicals. My yard was pesticide-free and there was no harm in putting petals on top of salads as a garnish or making a wonderful skin cream.

Did you know that the rose family includes some of the most delicious foods we eat? Apples, quinces, pears, peaches, plums, apricots, cherries, blackberries, raspberries, and strawberries all are members of the rose family.

After the plant blooms and petals wither and fall off, the wild rose produces a hip. These are tiny green fruits that develop during the summer and turn bright red in the fall. This plant reproduces by seeds, which are contained in the hip, and by forming new plants that root from the tips of arching canes that contact the ground. Birds feast on the hips, and as you can imagine, disperse the seeds over a wide range.

The wild multiflora rose has a small hip compared to its cousin, *rosa rugosa*. Another variety, *rosa canina*, is used in the supplement industry specifically for its high vitamin C content. However, the hip contains more than vitamin C, as do our wilder plants found in meadow or forest. The hip of the wild rose contains beta-carotene, bioflavonoids, phosphorus, vitamins A, B1, B2, E, D, and K.

I came across Euell Gibbon's research at the time I was observing the wild rose and her stages. He notes in *Stalking the Healthful Herbs* that the vitamin C content in one cup of hips is more than the amount found in ten to twelve dozen oranges.[29] During World War II, rosehip syrup was made in England as a source of vitamin C, as Britain was not able to obtain oranges, lemons, and other vitamin C rich fruits.

In the fall when the berries turn red, I gather a cookie sheet full of rose hips in the kitchen. I slice the hips in half to make drying easier. I place these cut hips on top of the refrigerator to dry – a dark place is needed. The hips tend to shrivel a bit when drying. Once dry, I place them in a glass jar and store in a dark cupboard.

To use the rose hips, I often add a small amount, maybe a half to one teaspoon, to herbal tea blends. They are quite bitter and the addition of spearmint or peppermint, for example, can help modulate the bitter flavor. Rose hips, with their high dose of vitamin C helps when we have a cold and are especially effective in herb teas with raw honey, peppermint, maple syrup, or even stevia.

I cannot talk about multiflora rose without mentioning invasives. This plant was introduced from the Far East. It can grow into dense thickets that out-compete other plants in the area, including natives. It has adventitious roots, meaning an arching cane can touch the ground and grow new plant from the leaf section. Wildlife, adventitious roots, and a vigorous perennial root structure give this plant three ways to propagate. As noted earlier, its perennial root system helps the land manage erosion. Like its cousins, the blackberry and raspberry brambles, these plants can be hard to remove if they take over a land space. In the meadow, I kept some, removed others, and observed the variety of wildlife that found refuge in my backyard meadow.

In loving the truth, the rose offers many lessons. Three ways to propagate says to me we have chances and choices about how to love. Growing where no other plant can grow says love is to be found everywhere even in the most difficult of times or places. Perfume from the blossoms holds the sweet scent of love's promise and beauty. Rose hips provide food, vitamins, and minerals for the cold season when most plants have died. The flowers themselves are esteemed and we "love" the color, scent, and the beauty so much that they are prized.

Roses have a long history. Wild roses are considered the very first roses some sources date back to seventy million years. They are also endemic to the Northern Hemisphere of our planet. Scientists have yet to figure out why that is.

Roses, in more recent history, lined nomadic routes and their petals were prized in bedchambers for a heady scent and for romance. They were symbols too and are well known as emblems of warring factions in England of older times. The first cultivars were brought to Europe from China in the 1800's. China's history of cultivation of roses goes back centuries.

Loving the truth is a challenge. To love another no matter the wrong or to forgive myself for knowingly or unknowingly inflicting hurt on another person or species becomes a lifelong quest, a hero's journey. Roses remind me of the beauty within and in the world. When I have stepped away from the truth in unconditional love my life gets thorny.

Love has many facets, many faces, some easy to know some hard to find. The rose then holds the paradox of "beauty amidst the thorns."

There is no way to hold something that is truly beautiful; not without consequences. There is a reason why roses have thorns.
—Adam Stanley

8. TEACH/SHARE THE TRUTH: GOLDENROD (SOLIDAGO CANADENSIS)

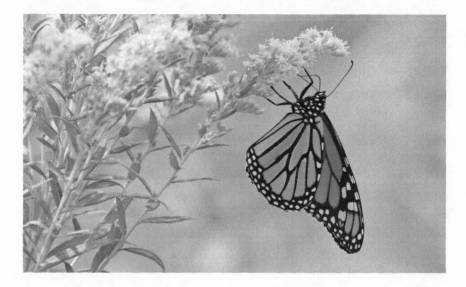

I enjoy teaching and sharing what I have gathered. Though not trained in education, I came to teaching through the back door and love the process. Years ago when I sat in circles with my elder brother Toe, he would make it very clear that he was not a teacher but that he would share what he knew. I always respected him for that. Today as I continue to explore Caroline Myss' work with archetypes, I have come to know the teacher as a role of mine.[30]

Today, I offer classes and give talks on wild edibles, those I learned from years in this meadow. Teaching is not simply public speaking, but preparing and synthesizing information in clear and concise ways to stimulate a student's understanding. The teacher is one who serves the truth by disseminating information known to be helpful and possibly healing.

I have come to know that the teacher, the teachings, and the students become intertwined, enmeshed, each a part of the other. In mythology, the rod or staff is depicted with various teachers such as Asclepius, considered the father of healing, and Moses, who brought laws to the Israelites.

The tall stalks/rods of goldenrod that fill the countryside with golden yellow color arrive with the close of summer. These flowers provide attractive, late summer sources of nectar for bees, flies, wasps, and butterflies, supporting 115 species.

My meadow areas with the spiral and medicine wheel paths hosted this amazing plant that brought amazing beauty. By August, the purple cone-flower was waning and Queen Anne's lace was turning to seed. To have the bright yellow color fill my backyard meadow felt like a gift.

In late afternoons, I would often sit in the meadow with a cup of tea. There, hearing the buzz of bees felt calming.

I cannot tell you the variety of bees that stopped by but there were plenty. It is only recently that I learned that this continent has over 200 species of bees and pollinators. At that time I had learned from an herbalist friend and beekeeper that the honeybee was introduced by colonists from Africa and Europe. However, I did not know the number and variety of bees that lived here prior to early colonization.

Goldenrod plays host for many beneficial insects and also repels some pests. Most of the 60 species of goldenrod are native to the U.S. There are a few species of goldenrod that are prized in Europe and planted in gardens, though it is considered a wayside weed here in the U.S.

North American tribes, such as the Cherokee, included goldenrod in their list of herbal medicines. They teach that goldenrod is an excellent wound healer, useful to alleviate the sting and inflammation in bug bites.[31]

Goldenrod is often accused of causing hay fever allergies. Yet the seed pattern does not seem to support this claim. The more likely culprit is ragweed *(Ambrosia spp.)*, which is often found in meadows and by road-sides in late summer and early fall like goldenrod. Ragweed disperses its seed into the wind, which can easily cause allergic reactions and irritations.

Ohio State University weed guide says the following regarding toxicity for goldenrod:

"None known. Goldenrods are often blamed for causing hay fever because they flower during allergy season. However, the true culprits are ragweeds (Ambrosia spp.). Goldenrod flowers are mainly insect pollinated, so the flowers are showy to attract insects and pollen is relatively heavy and sticky compared to ragweed. It is unlikely that the wind-blown allergens affecting hay fever sufferers include appreciable amounts of goldenrod pollen."

When I began to study this plant I came across the use of goldenrod in healing wounds. It has slightly astringent and antiseptic qualities that promote wound healing. This same property in tea form helps dry cold symptoms with mucus discharge. In Britain, it is one of the first herbs selected for upper respiratory catarrh, what we call the common cold. It can be blended with other herbs to help relieve flu symptoms.

My favorite preparation is to make a goldenrod infusion. It is one of the four plants I use to make my salve. It doesn't take much to fill a jar with beautiful yellow flowers and leaves. As with other plants where the flower is the primary ingredient, it is important to observe the blossoming time and pick plants at beginning bloom to peak bloom for potency. I pick a few stems with young blossoms. I strip the leaves and chop both leaves and flowers and store in a quart mason jar about two-thirds full. I add extra-virgin olive oil to the dry mixture and fill the jar to the top. The jar needs to be shaken one to two times per day to disperse the oil with plant mixture. Then I place the jar in a sunny location for five to six weeks, continuing to shake jar periodically. This is known as an infusion.

After the plant and oil infusion process is complete, I strain the oil and put the plant material back in the compost pile. The goldenrod infusion is now ready for use as a healing salve.

As our weather turned cold and with garden chores done, I would spend time in the meadow gathering the dried stalks of goldenrod for kindling.

The activity kept me warm as fall turned colder and helped me clean up the meadow space before winter hit. Goldenrod propagates itself by wind-dispersed seeds, though the seeds are heavy and sticky and thus pollinated by bees. It is also a perennial that sends shoots from its underground rhizome, a type of root. Gathering stalks used the leftovers that provided compost if left on the ground or kindling material. The end result was a cleaner space, less raking in spring, which allowed for new growth. Is this necessary in a large-scale meadow? I don't think so. Dead plant material creates compost for the soil. Did I have to do this in my meadow area? Probably not, but it helped in the springtime and gave me another use for this plant.

Goldenrods are wonderful companion plants, attracting beneficials and repelling pests, and their waving yellow blossoms bring beauty on hot summer days. In my meadow, their bright yellow flowers added contrast to the changing greens of the forest line that formed the back border off my property. Seeds of goldenrod can lay dormant in the ground for many years, and then under the right conditions, bloom again pushing forth golden rods that capture the sun, offering to share the truth of their medicine with us if we but ask.

For a time, several of us would gather in circle to share thoughts and ideas. My elder brother, Toe, a Narragansett elder, who was tall of stature, sat quietly before us sharing what he learned. The goldenrod, tall and beautiful, abundant in our meadows and fields, stands tall and quiet too. She has a rightful place among the healers of the meadow.

9. LIVE THE TRUTH:
POISON IVY (RHUS TOXICDENDRON)

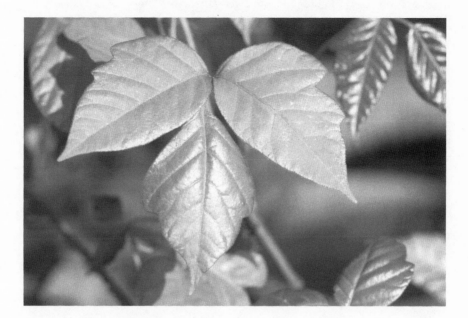

Loving the truth and living the truth are the two hardest places on the wheel. Both require us to overcome our ego's needs to be right and to step into a wiser understanding of self and the choices we make. The right use of will contained in "live the truth", for me means to understand my ego's messages so that I can hear the wiser part of me and then act and live from that place. It takes diligent practice and mindfulness to stay alert to the ways we fool ourselves. Living the truth from the inside takes courage and strength and even warrior fierceness may be required.

I don't know a gardener who likes poison ivy. Most of us are wary around it. I have met a few landscapers who seem okay working with it, meaning they seem immune to poison ivy's rash. I have also met some who are extremely sensitive to poison ivy's "poison" and have suffered severe reactions and needed hospitalizations.

While I have not needed to be hospitalized, I have had severe reactions to this plant.

My first encounter came from my contact with one of the "poisons" in our back woods at the home where I grew up. I say "poisons" because I am not sure if it was poison ivy or poison oak. Needless to say, for a nine year old, poison ivy's presence was quite difficult to handle. A body covered with itchy red rashes and swollen hands caused me to miss school for several days. The itch and discomfort were intense and hard to bear.

Later on in the home where I created this meadow, I naively cleaned flowerbeds under shrubs and a nearby tree, not realizing the dead branches I pulled out of the way were poison ivy vines. Rash quickly spread to arms and legs, and the itch was severe and uncomfortable, occurring in the peak of summer's heat.

At that time, I had begun studies with Robert Moss, a teacher of shamanic dream work.[32] This particular summer, legs and arms covered with pink calamine lotion and bandages, I attended a class of Robert's in a lovely retreat in upstate New York called Stillpoint. The simple cabins and meadows surrounded the teaching room and provided a natural and quiet setting for this work.

While dreams are not the subject of this book and shamanic practices in particular, I will say that we learned specific techniques for accessing dream time realms. The shamanic path offers a way to access other realms to bring healing for self and others, including accessing messages from the plant's spirit. In my path of understanding dreams through shamanic work, I learned an incredible detail about this plant not found in books.

In one of our shamanic journeys we were asked to focus on only one issue. I decided to focus on poison ivy. What could I learn about poison ivy if I could contact the spirit of the plant? This work could possibly take me beyond everyday facts. Could I actually do this and come back with a message?

Laying back, deep breathing, following the beat of the drum, I entered a deep inner place, an inner landscape I was comfortable with from previous practice and experience. I proceeded to imagine I was on a quest of sorts to understand this plant that caused such severe skin rashes and discomforts or worse.

Eventually as I relaxed, I saw myself at the base of a mountain outcrop. A huge plant was before me. I approached the plant cautiously noticing that it began to vigorously squirt its juices in all directions. It did not seem as if the plant was deliberately aiming at any one thing, but rather threw its juices out in any direction as it sensed my approach. Droplets were big and I was small so I crept carefully to avoid the large droplets, finding myself under its leaves, protected from the liquid onslaught.

In my studies as an herbalist, I was taught to approach plants respectfully. In this dream state, I knelt and offered a prayer of gratitude to this plant and felt the plant showed me quite graphically its abilities. We silently communed and I felt it informed me it was a warrior plant, a guardian and protector of the forest. It senses us long before we come near and shoots out its juices even if we don't touch it. The droplets are released to the air so some get poisoned in their lungs and eyes.

I was given permission to go forward and my "dream" continued to a visit with the spirit of the forest. I was moved and touched by this dream. When the specific drum beat sounded the call for us to return, I gave my thanks again before coming "back" into the room in the waking state.

What did I learn? Poison ivy seems to be a protector of the forest. In the Cherokee tradition, I learned that some plants are chiefs and warriors. It seems that poison ivy is a warrior plant of the forest, there to protect the forest and to inspire us to move carefully in and around the trees and plants of the meadow, forest, and our landscapes.

As our forests are being removed at an alarming rate, disrupting biodiverse ecological systems, this simple yet effective plant offers a timely message. Can we move in the forest more carefully? What are we removing from our landscapes? Can we work with the plants in our landscape differently? Can we commune with nature in some profound way? Can we really claim our co-creator role to be stewards of nature and all its elements rather than chop down rainforests or mountains with little regard for the consequences?

Those of us prone to these rashes want relief. Jewelweed, a common forest plant often found near poison ivy, is a common remedy to relieve or prevent the thick sap or juice of poison ivy from irritating the skin. I have found, and heard from other herbalists, that the best way to use jewelweed is to gather the fresh plant material and crush it. This will allow plant material to become moist in its own juices. This juice with plant material needs to be vigorously rubbed on the skin the same day of contact with poison ivy. After the rash has began and blisters erupt, jewelweed is not particularly helpful.

Homeopathically: *Rhus tox* is a common homeopathic remedy to help one develop some resistance to the rash. Many landscapers I met would use *Rhus tox* at the beginning of the gardening season to desensitize themselves from poison ivy's attack. Homeopathy is a specific system of preparation that uses plants and minerals that are extremely diluted. The theory is: like cures like.[33] For more information, please check the reference.

Poison ivy represents a forest protector. Instead of seeing it as a nuisance to be eradicated at all costs, I came away with a healthy respect for this plant and its place in our forest and landscapes. Respect to me means paying close attention when I enter a wooded area or working in a spot I am unfamiliar with. The early three leaves are easy to spot in early spring. It's in the summer I must be diligent in my efforts to identify this plant. In the fall, the leaves on the vines that wrap around trees are bright red and still easy to identify. Taking note when leaves are still on the vines, paying attention to which trees are wrapped in vines, makes fall and spring cleanup easier.

The lesson of poison ivy is one that I have passed on to others. Working in my meadow gave me the opportunity to care for nature's diversity in a simple backyard. When the neighboring children came to play, I set up guidelines. This place was a sanctuary. They were asked to respect the land and to not needlessly harm the plant life and critters that inhabited this space. My neighbors enjoyed the variety of flowers and the beauty of the backyard. Teaching the children to walk carefully was a duty I took on readily to honor and protect the presences in the meadow. At herbal gatherings I met several herbalists who are fierce warriors in terms of protecting at risk or endangered plant species.

Poison ivy's unconditional spirit of protection inspired me to respect it more and to be a protector here in my backyard.

10. WORK THE TRUTH:
DANDELION (TARAXACUM OFFICINALIS)

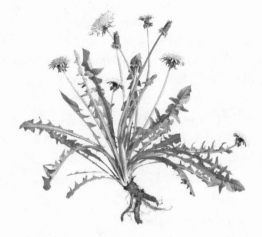

Work the truth concerns knowing our gifts and talents and sharing our creative gifts. Work can imply livelihood, toil, keeping on, effort, elbow grease, resolving a conflict, or creative pursuits made manifest such as an oil painting, a sculpture, a dance, a poem, a story. I associate this place on the wheel with my gifts and talents and ask myself: Am I using them to the best of my ability? Am I daring to share them and get out of the way with self-judgments? How am I expressing the gifts and talents given to me this day? These thoughts occupy me when doing the dishes, making a bed, arranging flowers, weeding, and pruning.

Dandelion, *taraxacum officinalis*, is a versatile plant and we are very creative in the use of the whole plant. Leaves and buds are a delicious early green in springtime. (I came across a recipe website with over 180 dandelion green recipes.) Flowers can be used in fritters, pancakes, cookies, and quiches, or to soothe tired eyes. Two of my students made a dandelion green cheesecake for a class project. Now that was an exercise in creativity that we all enjoyed. Roots dug in fall, when roasted, make a hearty coffee-like tea, brown and bitter. Dandelion roots aid in liver and gallbladder function.[34] Roasted dandelion root tea is delicious. This brew is a favorite of mine, and I find it worth the wait till the first frost of autumn hits the garden after which the roots can be gathered.

My backyard lawn in spring became a carpet of yellow flowers. Short and low to the ground, dandelions were prolific. We did not fertilize, nor were we experts on organic lawn growing. Consequently dandelions easily seeded themselves into our lawn. Many lawn fertilizers contain weed killers and since we did not use them our lawn was not "perfect".

It was always early spring when the first show of green leaves made their appearance. Most of the meadow and gardens still remained fallow. As spring took hold and buds formed on nearby trees, I found that the joy of spring was enhanced by these yellow blossoms dotting the landscape. Dandelions also grew in my formal gardens and I left most of them for fall root harvesting. In the meadow, they grew abundantly.

Dandelion greens are bitter. Our friends from Mediterranean areas use this green and know it well. Bitter is a flavor that has grown out of favor in America as we tend to choose salt, sugar, and fat, but bitter is important for our palate. The bitterness found in foods like dandelion greens stimulate our digestive juices. According to Ayurvedic medicine, the bitter flavor while not delicious in itself promotes the flavor of the other tastes. Bitter foods tend to be anti-inflammatory and cleansing to the liver. Because bitter is the antagonist to sweet taste, bitter foods/herbs are often given to people with diabetes.[35]

One doesn't have to wait for fall to enjoy dandelion tea. At our home in southwest Connecticut, I would often pull fresh dandelion greens, chop them, and then let sit in a glass of water about an hour before dinner.

This mild tea-like beverage can be strained and then drunk before dinner, another way to use the leaves and a practice that helps digestion.

In the spring I would gather dandelion greens and nettles and sauté the greens with garlic and olive oil, sometimes adding rice and goat cheese, or feta, for a hearty vegetable dish. Bitter yes, and more bitter as spring rolled in, but additions of cheese, rice, olive oil, and seasonings can tone down the bitter taste. In the evening, I gathered more leaves. Washed and finely chopped, these were a flavorful addition to the evening salad. The same finely chopped leaves are pungent and tasty additions to tomato sauce, soups, stews, or meat loaf.

About two years before I left the home in Connecticut where I tended this meadow, I attended a wilderness basic skills week in Maine. The highlight of the class was the wild food dinner we all helped prepare. The class took place in April and dandelions were obvious in the nearby fields. We gathered the buds found at the base of the plant, making these into a stir-fry, using onions sautéed in olive oil as our base, adding a little butter for taste to serve this as a side dish. The result was delicious.

Every morning our instructors made available a strong caffeine-free brew of dandelion roots. Bitter and coffee-like, without the caffeine, this became our morning cup o' joe. Not an everyday coffee drinker, I grew to appreciate the strong flavor and aroma of roasted dandelion tea. Roasted dandelion roots are often used as a substitute for coffee, along with chicory root, or barley, with honey, stevia, raw sugar, or maple syrup added for sweetness if needed.

Roasted dandelion root tea is easy to make, though time consuming. After first frost came, I would go out to my gardens to gather roots. Dandelions are easy to spot and with a small trowel are somewhat easy to dig up as they have a tap root. In gardens with good composted soil and no foot traffic, digging roots can be easy. After thoroughly washing the roots, I chopped them into coarse pieces maybe one-quarter inch long. (If you wait till after the whole root dries you will need an axe to chop them as they become that hard with the drying process.) Then I would place the chopped pieces in a thin layer on a cookie sheet.

The cookie sheets of dried herbs were placed on top of the refrigerator, a very warm place to dry herbs. After about a week, the roots were ready to be put in a coffee grinder. Then these coarsely chopped grains were placed back on the cookie sheet, spread out in a thin layer and roasted in the oven at 250 degrees. During the roasting process, I checked and turned the grains every fifteen minutes. After about one to two hours, the house smelled like roasted chocolate and coffee. Usually the grains were roasted enough by that time, turning a deep brown color. The sheets of hot grains were left to cool, then placed in a glass jar for storage. To use, steep one to two teaspoons of grain per cup hot water, or more, depending on how strong you like your brew, for ten to fifteen minutes, and then it will be ready to drink.

Dandelion flowers are edible, too. I added flowers to a quiche recipe. Quiche recipes today are easy to find. I started with simple ingredients: eggs, milk, and cheese, and then I might add a vegetable such as broccoli. Before placing the quiche in the oven, I would break apart dandelion flowers and sprinkle the petals over the top. They made a nice garnish. One or two flowers split apart add color, a bit of flavor without being overpowering to the overall recipe.

There are medicinal benefits to dandelion flowers. One pleasant use is to soak two to four flowers in warm water and then place on tired eyes for a pick-me-up. The stems when bent exude a milky substance that can help with skin blemishes such as acne. In the first herb class I taught to friends, I highlighted dandelions. I featured dandelion blossoms in pancakes, an eye wash, and teas. This first class gave me an opportunity to share what I had learned in fun and creative ways.

My herbal teachers often referred to dandelion as a tonic herb. Simply defined, it is an herb that nourishes and strengthens the body's systems. Dandelion is versatile, and the whole plant can be used. The root has a gentle cleansing action on liver and gallbladder. The leaves help reduce fluids, and its high potassium content helps lower blood pressure. Flowers can be mixed into dishes such as pancakes, fritters, and quiche.

The name "dandelion" is probably a corruption of the French "dent de lion", the tooth of the lion, since it was thought by many herbalists that the leaves resembled the teeth of the lion. Dandelion can be found scattered throughout the world, though the plant originated in Greece. Again, the early colonists brought dandelion seeds with them, and as you can imagine, they easily spread throughout North America. Today, the versatile and tenacious plant is frequently viewed as a detriment to lawns. They are subjected to tons of pesticides every year.

The dandelion has a firm hold in our landscapes. Seeds easily scatter in the wind. Hard to control and prolific, this hardy weed shows up most everywhere and is easy to find. They can be grown in a more controlled manner, which is popular in Europe. Johnnyseeds.com sells them by the packet. I would suggest dedicating a cultivated area in a garden for dandelion, for the versatile, delicious, and innovative uses possible with this most beneficial plant.

Creative work requires tenacity, to hold on to a vision, to carry on when our inner critic pipes up too soon. This little plant, one that seems to show up everywhere, demonstrates persistence. It is a powerhouse of nutrients, and we can and do prepare all parts of the plant in creative ways. So, keeping on when deadlines need to be met or hanging in there for just the right creative solution strengthens our resolution, our perseverance. Dandelion shares many creative gifts, inspires creative opportunities. As a tonic herb it strengthens all of our body's needs in holistic ways.

11. Walk the Truth: Mullein (Verbascum thapus)

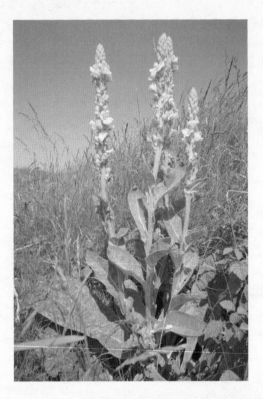

Walk the truth combines simple understanding with complex action. "Walking our talk" is a common phrase heard in Native American circles. What does that phrase mean to you? The folks I have met or read about that appear to stay true to their unique beliefs seem to have magnetism. I admire those who stand in their truth, no apologies. Walking the talk could be a code for leaders; to say what one means, to follow a promise; to be true to one's words in actions and deeds. For me, the true leader is one who has undertaken the inner journey, has put in the time and discipline to understand self in relation to the whole. Another facet of walking the truth can apply to the garden, the meadow, the forest. How does one walk in these areas? Do we needlessly trample, do we observe, what do we hear? Can we co-create with nature, choosing land sites more mindfully?

Perhaps an odd example in a book focused on the holistic and the natural, but *Star Trek, the Next Generation* in particular, is a wonderful model for right action as leaders in community. Its messages showed again and again how decisions and consequences governed strategic planning in facing seemingly insurmountable odds.

As we continue our walk along the wheel, at some point we will have to stand up for ourselves, to defend what we know as truth. Some of us may be called to lead and some of us may not. Walking our truth, standing tall in our center, seems to give off a magnetism, and that is what this place is about on the wheel of life.

With the meadow, as summer rolled in, I noticed certain wildflowers that showed up randomly in the yard brought in by the wind or fowl. Mullein rosettes began to appear one here and one there; not in any bed but by the house's foundation, the compost pile, or by the meadow's edge. Random plants, it seemed, found a home and took root. Mulleins are biennials, and thus it took me till the following season to understand their pattern.

The rosette is the first season's growth of mullein. Broad velvety, silvery green leaves look like an open rose that lies low to the ground. In its second year, mulleins produce a tall single stalk often three to five feet in height. This stalk's end produces small yellow flowers, as if a pinecone had blossomed. The flowers pop out throughout midsummer and are attractive to bees. The silvery, velvet leaves travel up the stem. Mullein leaves are often quite large, maybe twelve to fifteen inches long by three to five inches wide when a mature plant.

The leaf arrangement of the mullein is botanically interesting. Hairs thickly cover the leaves and give it a velvety feeling, while acting as a protective coat to the plant. Since mullein tend to be found in dry soils, this thickness of the leaf helps the plant from giving off too much moisture. The hairs also act as a deterrent to creeping insects and grazing animals, as they can set up an intense irritation in the animal's mucous membranes, encouraging insects and grazers to leave the mullein alone. While mullein tea is often recommended for coughs and colds, it must be strained before consuming as these tiny hairs can cause irritation to the mouth.

One of mullein's common names is "Candlestick plant". The downy hairs on the leaves and the stalks when dry make excellent tinder. When the plant has finished blooming, one can cut down the stalk, pour melted wax over the top few inches and create a torch. In the fall, I would cut down these dry stalks, as well as the dry goldenrod stalks, to make tinder for the fireplace.

One warm summer's day, when I still lived in southwestern Connecticut (I was still tending my own meadow at this point), I was out on errands and noticed a disturbed building lot in a nearby town. I had passed this way many times and noted that nothing much was happening. Empty and fallow, I began to notice the emergence of summer wildflowers. Eventually tall grey spikes of mullein caught my eye. One day I stopped and walked in. An unusual site greeted me. Several dozens of second-year mullein stalks formed a circle. Surprised and curious I walked around the inside.

My Native American friends had taught me to offer a prayer of thanks, leaving behind a pinch of tobacco before I picked anything. Silently I asked permission to pick some of the flowers. Mullein flowers infused in olive oil make soothing oil for swimmer's ear or can be rubbed on swollen glands. After giving thanks and feeling positive I gathered these bright yellow flowers here and there, always leaving plenty on any one stalk for the bees. I felt a joy and a connection to this "find". I walked in each direction and continued to pick flowers till I completed a circle. I did not strip these plants. Most were intact when I left. I gathered enough flowers to place in a small jelly type jar so I could make fresh mullein flower oil when I returned home. I gathered a few leaves to dry to keep on hand when winter came to have enough to brew a tea for a cough or a cold. The land was quiet. Two-year mullein stalks and flowers arranged by nature in a circle felt special. Yes the soil was disturbed and of poor quality. But seeing them standing tall, filled with blossoms, noticing how nature repairs soil and still offers us something in return, was indeed another lesson on my herbal journey.

Making a tea from the leaves is easy. Gather a few leaves, break into small pieces, and leave on top of the refrigerator to dry. When crinkly to touch, place in a glass jar and store in cool, dark cupboard for tea making. When making tea, place one to three teaspoons in your pot, pour boiling water into pot, and let sit for ten minutes. I used a thick towel or tea cozy to wrap my brewing pot. This keeps the tea warm for quite a long time. Remember to strain, as the hairs can be irritating.

Mullein flower oil is a useful infusion I have used many times.[36] As I mentioned, this is a good remedy for soothing an irritated ear canal. Please note: Do not place any liquid in the ear if you suspect a rupture.

Mullein flowers are bright yellow and often covered with bees found near the top four to six inches of the stalk. They are formed of five rounded petals, almost like miniature irises. The petals can easily be plucked off individually and dropped into a jar. To make the infusion, fill the jar about two-thirds full of blossoms, then add olive oil to the top of the jar. Cover and then let the jar sit on a windowsill to infuse. After five to six weeks, strain the flowers out and add them to the compost pile. I kept the oil in a clean jar, sometimes adding cloves of garlic to help relieve swimmer's ear type ear irritations, a frequent problem with my children. I found the best way mullein flower oil was helpful for this was to place the oil three to four times a day in the ear for three to four days. The oil is soothing. If any swelling, bubbling, pain persisted then we went to the naturopathic physician.

In Connecticut, naturopathic doctors are licensed to practice medicine. I found them helpful in relieving more serious symptoms.

Today, we are in a crisis of loss of biodiversity. Modern development for human habitation has decreased not only diversity of plant life but also diversity of wildlife that needs wild plants to survive. In many of our developed communities, we want flashy and long sustaining color, so wildflowers and weeds get yanked out. Unfortunately, we replace strong supporters of diversity with poor substitutes.

Second-year mullein is a repairer of nature and a strong source of food in natural habitats. It stands tall when winter comes. Though this plant may appear spent, its tall stalks that once displayed petite blooms harbor seeds that are accessible to sparrows and goldfinches. Insect larvae overwinter on these seed stalks and may provide a winter's food for flickers.

Although I tried, mullein do not like to be transplanted. Whether growing because of windblown seed or bird droppings, they seem to like staying put. I was not successful in transplanting them to other areas.

Mullein is a biennial and not native to the Americas. Today it is found world-wide. It escaped garden beds and became a part of our roadsides and meadow landscapes. Its first-year growth does not like to be transplanted. Its second-year growth puts up a stalk and petite yellow flowers. I left them where they showed up. I only removed them after the second-year's growth was spent and winter passed. The Native tribes here in the Americas used the roots too.

Walking the truth for me is demonstrated by living what we preach. I have taught respect for the natural world to my herbal and university students. I trusted my instincts to walk into the deserted lot. I came upon an unusual site. I gave thanks and asked before I took. David Winston, Cherokee Medicine Man and healer, taught me that when we approach the plant world in this way, the medicine is activated in a way that is hard to discern. The plants love it and simply give to us all they can for food, nourishment, medicine.

12. Give Thanks for Truth: Echinacea (purpurea, angustifolia, pallida)

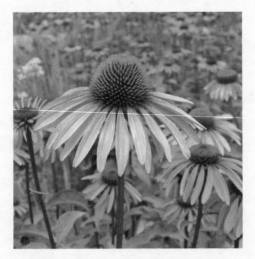

Number twelve on this wheel is about giving thanks. We could say "giving thanks for the truth". When I think of the twelfth position, like the clock, it sits up in the north part of the wheel, the place of elders. A true elder, as I learned, is one who shares their wisdom, who gives back to the community a perspective born of experience. Echinacea seems like an elder plant that has been the ambassador of the plant kingdom to the outside world. It seems this one plant became a favorite of those in the 1960s and 1970s, those folks who reopened the doors to herbalism after decades of being shut down. The early part of the 20th century, when traditional ways of herbalism were largely lost or ignored, favored the new pharmaceutical drugs hitting the medical scene. With the resurgence of natural medicine and holistic systems, echinacea was there lending itself to study, to exportation, to healing.

When I first began to cultivate the land and go to herb events/classes in New England, echinacea, the purple coneflower was always mentioned. It seemed as if the resurgence of using herbs for medicine was ushered in with the acclaimed healing benefits of echinacea. Herbalists from California to the east coast raved about this North American prairie native. I could not wait to plant these beauties in my gardens. At one of the gatherings, someone offered echinacea plants. I took a few home and planted them in my garden and watched them grow and propagate quite easily. I learned that the roots need to be in the ground for three to four years before the medicinal properties are at their fullest. So I watched again, made a note of the year I planted them, and observed how they increased in number and seemed to move in a counter-clockwise way. I did not plant them in the meadow area, but in a nearby garden.

Purple coneflower has become a favorite garden beauty for many reasons. It is a perennial that produces showy blooms that bees and butterflies love. Standing about two to three feet tall, it becomes a background plant that fills in a space with vibrant color and is a member of the aster family.

Herbalism lost ground during most of the 1900's when pharmaceuticals became our drugs of choice, but in recent years, as I noted earlier, there has been a resurgence of interest in the health benefits of plants. Purple coneflower in particular has been extensively studied for its effects on our immune system, and research demonstrates positive effects for resistance.

One study showed potential differences between two species of echinacea, the *purpurea* variety and *angustifolia* variety. It seems when *echinacea purpurea* was used in vitro (in laboratory) on the flu virus, it demonstrated a strong ability to neutralize the flu virus. *Echinacea angustifolia*, in the same laboratory study showed positive effects in neutralizing the rhino virus (the common cold).

The Sioux Indians used the root for snake bites and septicemia, a life threatening system-wide infection. When I first began my herbal studies, we were taught to use the root of purple coneflower for strengthening the immune system, to take a tea or tincture at the first sign of a cold. As more research was done in recent years, herbalists discovered that the whole plant has similar chemical constituents, and now you will find tinctures and herbal products listing the whole plant.

My first experiences with purple coneflower were to harvest the roots and make tinctures for family use. The common application at the time, which continues, is as a boost to the immune system in cold/flu season. My naturopathic physicians would frequently prescribe herbs for my children's cough or severe colds, and I noticed echinacea was often in the remedy. As time went on and as I used the herbal remedies more, my children seemed to be developing increased resistance to whatever went around the schools – the stomach viruses, pneumonia, colds. They usually had milder versions and were not knocked down, and missed fewer class days. The naturopathic physicians often recommended echinacea by itself or in a blend of herbs with echinacea included. In those years, I made more than I could use of echinacea tincture with the root, and often gave some of my supply away to family or friends who could use it.

In a prepared garden site where one does not walk on the areas where plants grow, digging for roots is somewhat easier. Dig the root after the flower is spent, wash thoroughly, chop into small pieces and let dry. Once dry you can place the dried and chopped roots in a coffee grinder and grind to a finer particle size. Echinacea roots, leaves and seeds all have a bit of a numbing quality when tasted. This quality is good to remember. I often reminded my students to note this quality, which is helpful when purchasing roots. Taste a bit and if a bit numbing you have good roots.

The chopped root can also be stored in glass jars and stored in a dark, cool closet for winter use. Roots typically take a little longer to steep, so I place dried roots into simmering water first, after ten minutes I added flowers and leaves, and then let steep another ten minutes.

The flowers of this plant are lovely and in my garden, its blossoms were covered with several species of butterfly: Swallowtail, viceroy butterflies, and common sulphur were frequent visitors. Echinacea is a "top ten" nectar source for these butterflies. The flower petals are good to eat and make a pretty garnish to a salad. I often pulled the petals apart to garnish the top of quiche, using only a bit as wild foods offer different textures and flavors, so a little goes a long way. Flowers and seeds can be added to vinegar. I have favorite vitamin mineral vinegar I make and purple coneflower seeds can be added to the recipe. Once a vinegar infusion sits for four to six weeks, it can be strained and kept in the refrigerator or in a cupboard for use for about six months.

As the 1990s ended, more research continued on the properties of echinacea and its effect on the immune system. Popular literature, fueled by the health food industry, claimed echinacea as one of the top natural remedies and preventives for the cold and flu season. Stems, leaves, flowers, and seeds were studied. Companies began including the whole plant in the tincture or dried herb products. When I apprenticed with Rosemary Gladstar in Vermont, she took us to an echinacea farm where the owner grew this beautiful purple prairie plant for commercial sale. Part of one field was harvested and placed in solution for shipping. Part of the crop remained as the owner rotated the harvest and replanted the harvested fields. Rosemary stressed over and over in her classes that the herb world did not need necessarily more product producers but rather more growers. This small local farmer took about two acres, planted *echinacea purpurea, angustifolia* in sections and then harvested them for sale to herb companies, organically grown, free of pesticides and fertilizers.

These plants are beautiful and grace any yard. They are American beauties native to our prairie lands. However they are also heavily exported, so please be aware of where your source of echinacea comes from. I recommend looking for organically grown as the product of choice. Research continues on this plant's properties and is often the first herbal remedy someone will try if they are new to holistic medicine.

Echinacea seems to be the plant that opens the door for one to explore herbal remedies. I have seen this happen many times as I worked in the health food industry. Echinacea, the purple coneflower, an ambassador, and a true emissary, opens the plant world to us when we are ready. I give thanks for the gifts of healing they offer.

13. BE YOUR TRUTH:
THE RAINBOW FLOWERS

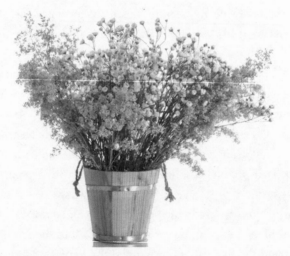

The rainbow is at the same time a bridge between the real and the unreal, the tangible and the intangible, as well as a door that leads into the world of imagination and fairy tales.
—Lama Anagarika Govinda, 20ᵗʰ-Century Tibetan Buddhist

The thirteenth place on the wheel is the center, the place where we run everything through our own truth. Some say our third chakra is an interface between our inner knowing and the outside world. The third chakra is near the center of our body, or the navel or solar plexus. "I have a feeling in my gut" or "a gut feeling" are common expressions.

I need "to sit with it first and then make a decision." Does it feel right or make me feel uncomfortable? "Follow your heart; believe in your dreams, where does you passion lie?"

These questions are a part of the wheel of life. At each place we are given clues, guidance, and support often through the third chakra. This place in our body, this connection, brings mystery and magic when we stay tuned to our inner guidance. This also helps us receive impressions, inspirations for life when in the natural world.

Changing my lawn into meadow became a truth for me. It was not done simply for my own enjoyment, though that was part of the truth. The land benefited: I created a small sanctuary in a small space that became a haven for a wide variety of wildlife. Others benefited: It was a place to teach children respect for nature in some measure. To do this, I followed my inner compass. I wanted to learn about which plants could heal, which plants offered sustenance, which would show up in my dreams, how I could help someone in distress. These plants showed me a variety of ways to accomplish all of these desires. Beautiful flowers, challenging roots, prickers, thorns, and grasses gave me a rainbow of opportunities to learn and grow season by season.

I began with the stories of my love for flowers and wildflowers. I would like to end this section on the plant wheel by remembering the flowers. Many of them are edible and, in small amounts, can garnish dishes, grace our tables, be added to recipes. Yellow-flowered dandelions, purple violets, purple and pink coneflowers, orange daylilies, white yarrow, yellow garlic or wild mustard, red clover, and the beautiful blues of mints – all of these can be used. (Always check before using.)

Color and texture creates a palette where nature fills in. Pure white "wild daisies" graced the meadow along with the dark yellow blossoms of black-eyed Susans, along with purple woodland asters, red and orange poppies, the pale pinks of fleabanes, yellow hawkweeds, purple violets, red raspberries, silvery mugwort, and white Queen Anne's lace. Bedstraw's tiny white baby's breath flowers hugged the outer edges of the meadow and created a lacy edge. Grasses waved in the everyday winds. Rainbows of light and color took various forms in the plant life and the insects and critters that inhabited this space. Simple, yet poignant life, radiated out my backdoor.

I did not know then that I would be writing this book to share my experiences of reclaiming land into habitat. Sitting with my deep desires of wanting to know more, honoring, then listening, observing, following inner guidance, gathering, drying, drinking teas, and studying herbals brought me to this knowledge I share with you.

For me, following a wheel spoke to me and guided me through a process of wonder and delight. This is the message and teaching of the thirteen. Listen and respond from that place within us of inner knowing and wisdom.

But this process was about more than personal pleasure. There is much at risk. Today speaks to an urgent need to reclaim land space, to create more habitats, to take care – or many of the species we know today will be gone tomorrow.

This wheel I have shared with you is my walk with the teachings. Each of us is unique. You can use a wheel, a mandala and create your own truths, however guided.

Rainbows hold magic and promise and like the iridescent wings of a dragonfly carry us to worlds beyond our imagination, hopes, and dreams. Rainbows tell us the storm is past. Rainbows delight all of us, that magical refracting of light into an array of colors, as if a gift from the sky.

THE NATURE OF OUR MISTAKES

THE VOICE OF NATURE SEEMS TO BE A QUIET VOICE; SOMETIMES IT'S SO QUIET I wonder how nature can be heard. Big issues, the problems of our world seem to clamor for attention incessantly much like street hawkers shouting, "This is wrong. No, come over here, look at this problem. Look at me, my problem is even worse." All of which overloads our senses.

The voice of nature is quieter than that, more subtle. Yet nature's voice is constant in the natural world around us much like the movement of the sun or the stars. It can be heard in the consistent hum of the bees. It can be seen in the magical weaving of a spider's web.

I have had the privilege in this lifetime to be in the stillness of a garden, a meadow, a land space where nature blossomed. Weeding, pulling dead leaf material out, pruning, raking, watching, and observing away from society's never-ending din. It is here in this subtle world of texture and form that I came to hear or sense the presence of nature and her guidance as I moved about, sat under my maple trees at the end of a day, and witnessed twilight's announcement of the coming night. I found peace, simplicity, connection, and appreciation for the beauty and the mundane.

I enjoy reading and this time in my life was no exception. I read voraciously, thirsty for more knowledge, more philosophy, more understanding of views on caretaking of the land, more understanding of spiritual development and the related study of herbology as known here in the West. I read about and was attracted to ancient Irish Druid love of the oak and their communion with the forces of nature. When I explored the Mayan culture or the Aborigine from Australia, I came across the same ideas. Even my journey into holistic medicine showed me that the ancient sages of each system whether Ayurveda, Taoist, Aboriginal, Ancient European, the Americas, held knowledge and wisdom in understanding the elements of nature. They also showed me what we do to one we do to the whole, the microcosm of man affects the macro-cosm, the Universe. These teachings seemed to have been brushed aside, lost not just with the onset of Christianity, but also with the onset of industry and technology where we began to devalue nature and her systems.

Some people have a knack for such perceptions and don't have to go through a learning process. That was not my case. I felt I needed to be more mindful of this innate ability we all have in order to bring more harmony into my life. The garden was a good place to practice. I watched, observed, learned much, prayed, and gave thanks as the meadowland unfolded season by season and then year by year. At first I decided to let the back area by the tree line grow, maybe eighty feet by sixty feet. We mowed a path in the middle and at the edges to keep land adjacent to ours neat and tidy.

Over that year and the next, I became more comfortable with following my intuition. I began to explore my inner world. Clairvoyance, defined by the Merriam Webster dictionary is: "the power or faculty of discerning objects not present to the senses." I began to have moments where I could see/know more than was outwardly present.

There are those who can see auras and who can read the energy field around a person. Some of these individuals came into my world, and in my encounters with them and in my acceptance of internal guidance, I dis-covered that I have some psychic abilities and more so, that most of us do. We are simply not trained or acknowledged in the use of these gifts, and we are told in Western medicine that such perceptions are "strange" or "delusional". This is not the case.

Feeling the energy, the presences of a garden can be done. We can trust that a simple knowing, a perception of a presence in nature is valid. Today, most of us are not taught these skills as we were taught in long forgotten times. But that knowing exists in our cellular makeup and can be activated with our intentions.

I did not believe this could be a part of my experience because on some level, I was insecure. I wanted someone to validate my experiences for me. But two events happened that changed my mind.

Sometimes we have the greatest learning through our mistakes.

Mistakes

Being with the land in my backyard was not a casual or fanciful endeavor. I truly wanted to have a connection with nature. I deeply wanted to learn about edible foods, and I wanted to give respect to the land. But I realized early on that I was alone here. My husband at the time would help with the mowing and digging. He was not interested in going further and understandably thought my ideas were quite fanciful, at the very least.

Due to an automobile accident, which caused a whiplash injury, my right shoulder needed care and attention. Repetitive activity, such as weeding or raking, needed to be done in short time intervals as I could not hold up longer. If my chores and routines with family aggravated my arm and shoulder, I had to pace myself differently, resting for a day or two before tackling garden chores.

Our soil was hard and rocky and digging proved difficult. However, once the garden areas were established, I found I could maintain them with ease. In the areas where I maintained control, mulch kept down the weeds.

Amazingly, the meadow itself, where I let it grow, needed very little maintenance. This was a gift. Pruning a few bushes here and there was relatively easy, and over time, the meadow became my focus, along with smaller side gardens. In these places I planted edible perennials. These small garden areas were approximately six by ten feet, a ten by twenty foot area, and a hemlock grove, with wild edibles on the outer edges with paths. These spaces were easier to maintain and held many types of plants that gave me plenty to harvest, dry, preserve, and utilize for family and friends and for the classes I began to teach.

My reading continued, and I came across these insights from Findhorn, specifically David, one of many touched by Findhorn's practical and spiritual demonstrations, who described experiences with the plant spirits they referred to as fairy and devic realms and their message to us:

> *"If in the process of the experiment we are hurt through injurious actions to the forms we build and minister to, we will have patience and bear the hurt, knowing that you are learning."*[37]

Despite my reading and my openness, at this time I did not see fairies and Devas, but felt their presence, which sometimes left me frustrated.

As I mentioned before, I read extensively in this period of my life and enjoyed others' stories about their experiences with nature presences, all somewhat different from mine but all with a central thread of understanding.

I want to stop here for a moment to say these experiences of others are valid. This was also a part of my learning at that time.

There are many ways to connect with nature, and it has taken me a long time to validate and understand my journey. Your journey and your process may be different.

In other words, do not invalidate your own experiences just because they may be different from others. "Seeing" was a big deal to me back then. If I did not see these wee folk, as the elders called them, then in my perception, I was not connecting to them. That is not true, as I later learned.

However you feel you are working with nature, understand it is valid. We are connected, and whether you see or hear them, or not, they know us. It took me till the end of my journey with this land and my leaving, before I really understood how connected I had become to this small suburban backyard space and the nature presences that governed it.

During this period of transformation, two incidents brought home my change in understanding and my new perceptions of our connection to nature.

My sons loved to play ball with their neighborhood friends. While we had a large backyard, the meadow on the left encroached on some of that space. My son and his friends wanted more room. I sat with my family, discussing this, and reluctantly agreed. But I had not sat with the meadow before my husband got the lawnmower and cut the meadow back. In this process, he took more than we agreed.

When the deed was done I walked back through the meadow, saddened when I realized how much of the meadow had been cut back. Then it was as if I heard moans, cries of pain, agony. I cannot describe how it felt in that moment. I found myself grieving. I did not know at this point how connected I had become to the presences here. For days I went out and apologized deeply from my heart. I had a connection to the meadow that I did not fully understand although I knew at the time that this earth needs to be respected.

The Native American teachings gripped my heart. I walked countless times with tobacco for morning prayers and cornmeal at night, as I wandered around the yard giving thanks.

These daily acts kept me in communion with the presences here. The message David from Findhorn received hit home. I opened the door with my intention to connect with them. They responded. However I truly did not understand that we can hurt them if we discount the validity of that connection and just randomly "cut" into these realms without mindfulness and checking in with them. This is done in a whisper, a prayer from the heart as communication tends be on the intuitive level.

The second experience occurred later on in the fall.

Saturday morning rolled around like many others. We were doing chores.

To give context, understand that every day I would sit in my meadow in the morning, harvest plants before noon, wash, dry, and preserve plants by supper. Through this routine, I developed a deep connection and commitment with this space. We had beautiful established trees on the property, and I had named the trees – or accepted their names, depending on your perspective.

In my travels with my Native American elders and in my work with herbalists and my time spent in meditation circles, that I have only briefly mentioned, I learned that nature was full of presences that were/are intimate and personal. Grandmother would say, "Brother Wind is strong today. The Earth Mother, our Mother is full of curves, just look at the mountains and hills."

My elder brother would say, "Brother Fox showed up today." My meditation teacher would have us name all we are and what we experienced in our spiritual work. So I gave my trees names. It felt connected; it felt personal. I addressed them when I sat beneath them and when I walked around giving thanks. They were real presences to me, whether any believed me. And believe me, most folks I knew back then would not have accepted this knowing. But to those acquaintances I met in Native American circles, this knowing was no big deal.

The beautiful maple in the front yard outside the living room bay window was named Theodore. I would sit from time to time in my living room, often at night after my sons went to bed, in its presence. This particular Saturday morning I was in the house doing laundry when I felt something was wrong. I was not sick and the house was quiet. Puzzled and feeling as if I was uncomfortable in the gut, I went outside to where my former spouse was doing yard work. He had been mowing. I walked out and asked him what he had been doing.

After a short discussion, he said he had cut a low branch from Theodore, the large maple in our front yard, as it was in his way. My former spouse is a good man, but he simply had no interest in nature as I did and did not understand what troubled me. He could not understand my connection or the pain I felt, as if the hurt had happened to me too. Again, given our culture's focus on the tangible, logic, and reason, this was understandable. Working on the intuitive level and trusting a connection, guidance, perceptions are simply not taught in our culture.

Can we prune, mow, and chop trees and shrubs? Yes. However, I learned that when stating my intentions to nature, specifically show me how we can work together, I had to realize I got answered. If I took the communion seriously, then I had to take responsibility for warning them when lawnmowers came out, asking and then listening for when and if it was time to prune. This shows respect.

I cannot change another. I spoke to the land and told them what I could do for them and not do. And I hoped they would understand our different approaches, in some measure. Though I could not articulate it as well as I can today, it was real. Also to cut and prune is okay. However when I opened to nature's presence, I could feel the consequences of actions. These two examples hit home about a responsibility to commune with nature first. They easily comply, but like you and I, they appreciate being asked first.

Most of us are cut off from nature's presence – or we choose to be cut off because we do not know what exists. All I can do, and could do at the time, was do my best to honor the connections as I felt them. I warn them when I am coming to harvest, prune, dig, weed, etc.

In 1998, I taught an herbal intensive program. This was the year before I began to teach my first Holistic Health class at the local university. My students and I met one Saturday per month from May to October. During this class, I taught my understanding of walking the land with respect, teaching these wonderful folks to give thanks before taking. They learned about wild edibles, how to make tea and decoctions, lotions and creams.

When we held our wild food cooking class and they had to gather from the meadow to make a salad, my heart expanded. I watched them gather plants that day with respect and loving kindness. I sensed they got it. It made the journey worthwhile. These experiences deepened my understanding that I in fact had a connection with this land and helped me to understand what I would need to do when it came time to leave this property.

FRUIT: SEVEN EASY STEPS FOR TURNING A LAWN INTO MEADOW

Meadows are grasslands found in forested regions – the open patches of grasses and wildflowers common to the Eastern forests, the montane forests of the Rocky Mountains, and the Sierra-Cascade ranges, and the Pacific Coastal forest.
—Landscaping with Wildflowers and Native Plants, p. 59

MY MEADOW DID NOT REQUIRE MANY STEPS. I LOOKED AT THE GRASS IN THE BACK quarter acre by the tree line and realized I had many common medicinal and edible species, which tells you my soil was not great. Many of our common weeds, as mentioned in previous sections, are soil stabilizers, soil builders. They often give a clue as to the state of the soil.

After living at this home for a couple of years, we made the decision to let the grass grow. After about two seasons, I made careful note of which plants came and went, and which plants, like perennials, goldenrod and yarrow, claimed some permanent residence. As mentioned earlier, these plants became my teachers in very practical ways.

Meadows require some planning, depending on purpose, types of flowers, topography, and the growing zone.

For those of you who would like practical guidelines on creating a meadow, whether reclaiming a flower bed, or looking at unused pasture land, and/or everything in between, the following will be helpful.

I have highlighted seven "how to" steps for creating a meadow. Before discussing these steps however, I would like to focus on the importance of soil:

Soil is probably the most complex ecosystem on earth. It has physical and chemical properties, structure, and integrity and a single handful may be home to more than a billion organisms.[38]

This earth matter, called soil, grows living organisms. Most of these amazing populations can be viewed only under a microscope. Soil organisms flourish when the soil is in good health. They convert organic matter and minerals into the vitamins, hormones, disease-suppressing compounds, and nutrients that plants require to grow.

Soil is a mixture of mineral particles, organic matter, water, and air. A handful of soil is about twenty-five percent water and twenty-five percent air. Both are needed for the organisms to thrive and complete their tasks of conversion mentioned above. Plants get nitrogen, an essential nutrient, from the air.

Organic matter is defined as the soil material that remains after most decomposition has taken place. Another way to describe organic matter in soil is humus. Humus is a brown or black complex material resulting from partial decomposition of plant or animal matter and forms the organic portion of soil.

The documentary *Dirt: The Movie* reminds us that, "God did not give us this amazing dirt to mistreat it." The movie highlights our relationship to the soil. Many folks interviewed in the movie were/are passionate about reclaiming the soil.

More important is that as humans we have a choice: to work with nature or against nature.

Working with nature brings benefits. Natural fertilizers enrich the soil. Enrichment is the key word because this concept and application give back the nutrients needed to grow our crops.

Over and over, from research scientists in the lab to those with a long history of farming, all know there is a language to the soil. But much soil has been lost or degraded – we have lost a third of our topsoil in the last 100 years.

Pesticides deplete the soil on all levels. Mono-crop farming needs excessive amounts of nitrogen. Excess nitrogen flows into streams and oceans creating super weeds that mean a dead zone for local fish and algae populations by increasing the amount of nitrous oxide in those waters.

Meadows can repair soil, provide habitat, support ecosystems being depleted today. Some plants such as multiflora rose and yarrow can prevent erosion and further loss of topsoil. Meadows do not require pesticides or herbicides to maintain as the variety of plant life brings in a balance. Meadows only need water to start seeds, and after that, they are on their own.

Michael J Rhodes reminds us in his book, *Conscious Gardening*:

"Care for the soil with conscious attention. Be aware and conscious of the soil as a living medium. The soil is alive and it is your responsibility as a conscious gardener to support and value that life. It is estimated that the weight of life in the soil far outweighs the weight of all humans, animals, and creatures that live on the soil. That is a sobering thought. It is up to us, as conscious Beings, to support this natural balance, in however small a gesture, by the care and intelligence of our actions in the garden."[39]

Step 1: What is your purpose? Will your site fulfill your purpose?

Most of us want glorious, ever-blooming color from spring to fall. But gardens and meadows require patience. Perennial mixes will not bloom the first year as they send deep roots, but the result the second year is worth it. They will produce over the next few years. Native grasses provide texture and subtle color. They help keep weeds down.

When planning a meadow space, some important questions to ask are:

1. Where is the site I want to change or create in regard to property lines?

2. Are there any easements, setbacks, zoning regulations, right of ways that I need to consider/be mindful of before tilling?

3. If there are no restrictions and the site supports sun and water requirements, then measure the plot size so that this can be used for seed calculations.

Step 2: Site Evaluation

1. Location. Is it sunny? Wildflowers need a minimum of six hours of full sun.

2. Is the space near the forest? Remember the forest will move in. Mowing needs to be considered. How easy will it be to mow this site?

3. Is the meadow on a slope? Can you mow the slope or will you have to weed and maintain it by using a hand weeder or by hand?

4. What is the area at the bottom of a slope like? Will there be pooling of water in spots?

5. Type of soil available. Wildflowers are hardy, but it never hurts to get a soil sample first. Local State Agricultural Extension Services provide soil sample test kits at reasonable costs. Poor soil may require more seed. How much rock is present?

6. Is the area out in the open and dry and well drained?

7. Are you reclaiming lawn and/or planting islands of wildflowers in your yard?

Step 3: Soil Preparation

Taking a soil sample first will give you an analysis of soil quality. Poor soil will require more seeds, and the sample results can give the type of amendments you could apply if necessary. Compost mulch can be turned into the soil after it is tilled. Wildflowers are hardy plants, often drought resistant.

Tilling the soil helps remove weeds, creating a fresh start. Let sit for two to three weeks and then till the new growth again. This can be repeated a third time before planting wildflower seed. Most garden sites recommend shallow tilling as you can disturb dormant seeds in the soil with deep tilling.

Step 4: Fertilizers

Many garden centers recommend herbicide applications after the first tilling when the subsequent first shoots come up. Synthetic fertilizers denature soil and deplete the soil in the long run, and I do not recommend them. Wildflowers in general are hardy, tough, and resilient. Fertilizers will encourage weeds and grasses.

I would like to comment on Roundup, a common herbicide recommended by garden centers and extension services.

Nature is intelligent. There is a pattern and reason to our natural world. Bugs, birds, and other wildlife can help our gardens grow. I have heard many stories over the years about home organic gardens that thrive without the use of synthetic fertilizers and pesticides. In my garden I noticed that the Japanese beetles munched and defoliated spearmint leaves but the garden vegetables were not overrun by them. I ask these questions: Why are we choosing to turn a blind eye to the toxic effects from pesticide residues that exist in our current world? Why are other countries ahead of the U.S. in research and the sharing of that research to lawmakers when we know, and the lawmakers know, of the potential toxic effects to humans, animal and insect populations as well as our precious soil?

It is my intention to stay the course and ask you to question the plants you choose, the land that we could disrupt, and to change course if something tugs at you; if something does not feel right with the incessant application of toxic material to our natural world.

Jeffrey Smith, from the Institute of Responsible Technology, states:

> *"Roundup acts as a chelator of vital nutrients, depriving plants of the nutrients necessary for healthy plant function ... destroying beneficial organisms that suppress disease causing organisms and help absorb nutrients ... Interfering with photosynthesis, reducing water use efficiency, shortening root systems and causing plants to release sugars with changes to the soils pH ... Stunting and weakening plant growth ... Promoting disease-causing organisms in soil, which then overtake the weakened crops ..."*

Smith presents emerging studies that show what Roundup does to the soil.

In *Conscious Gardening* by Michael J Roads, the author reminds us of the value of soil.[40] Soil is at the heart of nature and our world, whether food, lumber, habitat, clothing etc. Natural fertilizers enrich the soil. Synthetic ones denature and deplete the soil. This simple principle is easy to demonstrate and understand. Mr. Roads offers many natural ways to fertilize that he personally uses. Books are plentiful on the subject of organic farming, creating compost and mulch with natural soil enriching materials.

Studies emerge daily that warn us of the detrimental effects pesticides have on our health and on the health of our children.[41] University ecology clubs, among others, have some institutions pulling weeds by hand, diminishing or eliminating toxic fertilizers and pesticides.[42] These campus groups are working hard to make campus lawns safer. Elementary schools are putting in their own gardens and using these harvested foods in their cafeterias.[43]

Other studies relate concerns health care professionals have about allergies. Some physicians are advising their young patients to remove genetically modified foods from their diets. Animal studies show damaged sperm cells, altered DNA functioning, sterility.[44] These effects can come from seeds that are injected with systemic pesticides such as Bt or Roundup.

Beekeepers across the globe are concerned about the possible link of crop pesticides affecting the health of bees and their link to Colony Collapse Disorder. Europe has made a connection between systemic pesticides genetically placed in crop seeds with the decline of bee populations and some European countries have passed legislation to ban certain systemic seeds.[45]

Why are we behind? Why are we afraid to explore other possibilities? Nature is so abundant. Can you count the leaves on every tree, every grain of sand? Did you know that every seed has the potential for producing a million more? It is my feeling we have an abundant creative universe to co-partner with. All we have to do is ask.

Obviously I do not advocate the use of pesticides on meadowland. The very idea of a meadow and its diversity allows nature to manage its own check and balance. It encourages wildlife and supports many species. I am not one to study bugs, but I wish now I knew the names of the different species of bees that visited my meadow. I saw species I had no idea existed before this adventure began. Dragonflies come in a rainbow of colors. Butterflies big and bold, tiny and purposeful, added a grace. Spiders kept vigilant patrol and many unseen organisms added to the balance.

My meadow may not have been as pretty as some of the garden books. I did not seed consistently and that was deliberate. But there was a carpet of canary yellow blooms, purple violets, and silver rabbit's foot. My neighbors liked the profusion of flowers. Their children played here and were respectful of nature here. I reaped the benefits being in the stillness, the magic, and the beauty that our poets extol when writing about nature.

Step 5: Sowing Seed

Once you have completed your last tilling of the ground area, plant immediately. When we sow right after tilling, we give new seeds a chance to sprout. Sowing can be done by hand.

1. Mix four to five parts of sand with one part seed. Place mixture into two pails. Note: Sand dilutes the seed so you can sow more evenly. It is light colored and can be easily seen over dark turned soil allowing you to track where you have been.

2. Take one bucket and disperse seed in opposite directions, for example, east to west. Take the second bucket and sow the seed in opposite directions, north to south.

3. Once done, gently tamp down the seed. You can use an empty lawn roller or a board to walk on to gently compress the seeds. Remember some seeds are so tiny that too much soil cover can prevent seed germination.

4. Do not rake or cover area.

Step 6: Water

Keeping the ground moist will help seedlings grow to about six to eight inches high. At this height they have the ability to thrive without consistent watering. They should be okay unless drought conditions prevail. During a drought some plants will naturally decrease flower production. Remember many of these plants help prevent erosion.

Step 7: Maintenance

1. Mow one time/year after killing frost; this helps disperse seed and decrease brushy growth.

2. For small areas that may show unwanted plants, you can remove them by hand and then reseed that particular spot. For large areas, one can retill the affected area and then reseed following guidelines stated above.

3. Leave clippings as this becomes your "natural" fertilizer.

The first year can be the most "work". Once done turning lawn into meadow, maintenance is easy, uses little water resources, decreases mowing, and eliminates the need for synthetic fertilizers, pesticides.

The end result is rewarding.

SEEDS: SEEDS OF CHANGE
AND GOODBYES

Life does not accommodate you, it shatters you. It is meant to, and it couldn't do it better. Every seed destroys its container else there would be no fruition.
—Florida Scot Maxwell

IT IS CHALLENGING TO DESCRIBE THE SUBTLE, MYSTICAL EXPERIENCE OF TENDING THE land. I spent hours walking, harvesting, digging, pruning, listening, enjoying the simple beauty that existed here, during the twelve years I tended to this backyard land space. I observed the growth pattern for appropriate harvest time; which parts of the plant to use and which type of preparation I would use in everyday application. During those years I dreamed of medicine wheels, animals, insects, birds, and reptiles that stimulated me to keep on digging into myself, to keep on drying herbs, and making tea, tinctures, or salves, and later to use them in acknowledgement of the healing gifts these plants offer.

Nature is not perfect. Sweating is okay, and sometimes we need a sting or two to get our attention. I lost my fear and hesitation of stepping off the medical model I was taught. And though I value the education and experience of it, I learned there is much to be gained with simple measures. I share and continue to teach today from this place of experience and wisdom. I create bridges of understanding between both worlds, the allopathic and holistic models. This little meadow, in a suburban backyard, provided the opportunity as I listened to a prompting from my deep within.

Spring's arrival at the turning of the seasonal wheel means winter's dormant period ends. This enchanted me each year. Luscious green leaves filled with sunlight punch surrounding hillsides and meadows with vibrant color much like an artist who first tackles the background on his canvas. When the flowers burst in a rainbow of color in summer I felt at peace. I sat next to my trees and pondered decisions I would soon need to make. I admired bats' single-minded purpose, gathering mosquitoes on their evening rounds. I walked the perimeter giving thanks many a night. I awakened some mornings and strolled through the wet grasses. Autumn's harvest and bounty were treasured gifts when winter's emptiness took over the land. I walked the land when frozen too, when the land was fallow, grasses spent and brittle, and appreciated the cycles of nature.

Being present takes diligence. The meadow became a daily focus. I learned more over the years that complimented and added to the learning from the books I love. Tenacity and patience, a stubbornness born out of a desire to be in partnership with nature, the earth, fueled the will to carry on.

But change comes. Nothing stays still. Life pushes and pulls us in new directions, like the yarrow that began in the east but moved to the north the next season. Storms blew in and the winds of change howled. I knew as my marriage fell apart I would be moving away. I also knew from the discussions I engaged in with elders and others in those circles that I needed to leave this land space in a sacred way.

I set wheels in motion for this move to take place. Divorce is never easy on anyone and takes time. I continued to take care of this place till my divorce became final, and I began to pack my bags. Regrets? Some, however I made a commitment to myself to take a chance to feel a part of me beating again. I wanted to continue the "soul" work I discovered through dreams. Listening to the deeper self is a part of that journey. If I received a message to not go somewhere or to be with a certain person, I listened.

There were times when I was warned and times when I got the go light. I often dreamed of my teachers and felt the learning and connections go deeper than ordinary reality. The feeling to leave came in not only on the gut level, but also through my dreams, so strongly, no matter how I prayed.

It is a part of life. Just as with the seasons, some relationships wither and die and fall away. Autumn's dance of the falling leaves reminded me to "let go and let God."

I wanted to leave the meadow in a good way. I knew that if this was right for me it would be right for all involved. I had children to account for and I wanted them to see their mother as a woman who thoughtfully faces her fears and lives her dreams. I wanted them to see two parents make decisions that were for the best.

I tended the meadow for twelve years, and at the end of this time, I knew big changes were on the horizon. Was I doing the right thing? Could I make it on my own through the myriad of changes before me? These thoughts crowded my nights and pestered me during the day.

When boxes were packed, contracts close to signing, I went into the meadow one morning and sat in the silence. I brought sage and tobacco and began my prayer ritual. I set my intention of saying goodbye and expressed my deep gratitude for being able to care take this space. I said goodbye with tears and some regret. The perpetual question, "Was I doing the right thing?" was asked again, though by now I had the answer and plans were in place. Again, however, I was concerned for the meadow and all that lived there. After all, I had set the land up as a sanctuary but could no longer care take this land.

"Yes," they whispered. *"We'll be fine. So will you."*

I saw them standing there in the back left of the meadow looking at me. Men and women, animals standing in the near distance like a mirage. I felt that "they" came to send me off, to acknowledge my goodbye. I so wanted the presences here to feel my gratitude for their patience with me as I stumbled through a learning odyssey. The plants, well, we simply got to know one another here as their slow and subtle whispers filled my heart and spirit. They spoke to me in a cadence of patience and timelessness. But I had to leave, to move on into a new beginning, a new journey. Their presence acknowledged my simple ceremony of ending in its purity.

A few days later before I left for the last time, I went out into the meadow to reconnect. I was feeling saddened and happy – a paradox of feelings. As I said my prayers and sat quietly, I could not connect with the energy I was so familiar with. This space felt empty. Oh, I felt the wind blow through the grasses and the bees stilled hummed. The sun moved through the sky.

I realized that I had many doubts along the way of connecting with nature, those presences defined by Findhorn and others, as this meadow-land developed. This day, knowing my departure was a few days away, I finally knew differently.

This place and I experienced a communion of sorts over the years. However on the day I chose to say goodbye, I noticed the wind blew much like the breezes that blow tumbleweeds around a ghost town. The space felt empty. "They" were gone. I could not feel "them".

In the far distance up in the sky it seemed I saw a bubble of light, large and commanding, move away. I felt an intelligent presence waited for me to leave, to say my final goodbye, and then it was gone.

This meadow was my journey into nature, its essence and mine, soul if you will. I needed to say goodbye one last time to experience the leaving of some-thing far grander than I could have ever imagined or known was possible.

In the way of all true seekers I closed one gate and opened another, one filled with the wonder of new beginnings, new discoveries. I hoped faith and trust would be my companions as I decided to travel a different path through a new garden I was eager to discover.

It was in the leaving that I came to understand how much we shared, how much I was taught even though I thought at times that nothing went on. Yes, they sprouted, grew, blossomed, and died, some leaving seeds, some springing to life again.

It was the communion, the knowing of connecting to nature's presences that govern the plant kingdom's realm that was surprising.

Findhorn reminded me of the deep connection we have through our intuitive senses and to know that when we ask we receive.

I learned that day that I could not go back. They took me at my word.

At the Garden's Gate is born from these experiences. How can I use my gifts, my talents and contribute more deeply? Here I am today writing the story, a simple tale of medicine wheels and plants that contributed to and supported diversity in the land and growth within myself.

Today our land spaces are dwindling. Animals are severely endangered.

Today, years after the Vietnam War, Dow Chemical Company is seeking to replace Roundup, a pesticide used in agriculture, with napalm, 2,4-D. The extensive use of Roundup over the past two decades has produced super weeds, immune to Roundup's application. Many of our veterans, the Vietnamese as a people and a country suffered from the use of this substance. Yet today it's back on the marketplace and Dow seeks to use it on our crops.[46]

Researchers like Dr. Stephanie Seneff, at MIT are proving how toxic these chemicals are to our biology.[47] It's appalling to me that though we protest, our lawmakers are approving the use of 2,4-D in and on our crops. Many sources "have established links between 2,4-D exposure and birth defects, hormone disruption, and cancers like non-Hodgkin's lymphoma." (Pesticide Action Network of North America).[48]

These two products alone are contributing to soil damage, pest resistance, and antibiotic resistance as antibiotics are contained in Roundup for genetic insertion into plants and the product sprayed on the ground.

The time to act is now; to sign petitions, let our lawmakers know where we stand. Connecticut and Vermont have passed legislation, beginning steps to guarantee our right to know. Growing our own meadows, gardens for food or habitat contributes to the overall health of all of us not just corporate bottom lines.

With focus we can reclaim lawn, no matter the size, and replant. There are many edibles like blueberries, loganberries that can be planted in our landscapes quite easily and contribute food for humans and other species alike. Meadowland with its rich diverse makeup contributes greatly to healing soil and providing sorely needed habitat.

Seeds have the potential to produce a thousand more. And each of those thousand, thousands more, and so on.

We can let nature help, and above all, we can work with nature with respect and communion.

At the Garden's Gate is my seed that I choose to plant in the outside world. I hope it carries inspiration and seeks to be a voice, a reminder for our evolving consciousness, that we and nature are one.

ENDNOTES

1 Weed, Susun, S. 1989. *Wise Woman Herbal, Healing Wise.* Woodstock, New York: Ash Tree Publishing.

Roads, Michael, J. 1987. *Talking with Nature.* Tiburon, California: H J Kramer Inc.

Wright, Machaelle Small. 1987. *Behaving as if the God in all Life Mattered.* Jeffersonton, Virginia: Perelandra.

2 Allopathy defined: The treatment of disease by conventional means, i.e., with drugs having opposite effects to the symptoms.

3 Naturopathy defined: A system of alternative medicine based on the theory that diseases can be successfully treated or prevented without the use of drugs, by techniques such as control of diet, exercise, and massage.

4 http://blogs.ei.columbia.edu/2010/06/04/the-problem-of-lawns/ Lakis Poycarpou wrote this article for the Earth Institute.

5 Arguelles, Jose 1987. *The Mayan Factor.* Santa FE, New Mexico: Sun Bear & Co.

6 Bear S. and Wabun. 1980. *The Medicine Wheel.* New York, New York: Prentice Hall Press.

Brook Medicine Eagle. 1991. *Buffalo Woman Comes Singing.* New York: Ballantine Books.

Beverly Hungry Wolf. 1982. *The Ways of My Grandmothers.* New York: Quill.

7 "The Findhorn Garden Story", 4th edition, by the Findhorn Community
© 1975 by the Findhorn Foundation;
published by Findhorn Press, Scotland Findhorn Community.

8 Wright, Machaelle Small. 1987. *Perelandra: Garden Workbook*.
Virginia: Perelandra, Ltd.

9 Dyer, Dr. Wayne. *The Power of Intention*. United States: Hay House.

10 Moore T. 1992. *Care of the Soul*. New York, New York: HarperCollins
Publishers, Inc.

11 Sams J. and Nitsch T.1991. *Other Council Fires Were Here Before
Ours*. San Francisco.

Freesoul, John Redtail. 1991. *Breath of the Invisible: The Way of the
Pipe*. Wheaton, Ill. USA: The Theosophical Publishing House.

12 Fincher, Susanne F. 1991. *Creating Mandalas for Insight, Healing
and Self-Expression*. Boston: Shambala.

13 Andrews, Ted. 1993. *Animal-speak*. St. Paul, Minnesota.
Llewellyn Publications.

Sams & Carson.1988. *Medicine Cards*. Sante Fe, New Mexico: Bear
& Company.

14 Estes, Clarissa Pinkola. 1992. *Women Who Run With the Wolves*.
New York: Ballantine books. P. 236-237.

Myss. Caroline. 2002. *Sacred Contracts*. New York: Three Rivers Press.
P. 123-134.

15 Faraday, Ann. 1990. *The Dream Game*. New York: Harper & Row.

Garfield, Patricia. (1992) *Creative Dreaming*. New York:
Ballantine Books.

16 Myss, Caroline. Myss.com. She has list of talks, lectures, newsletters.

17 Montgomery, Pam. No book available from Pam at this time. Hands
on type of class. Visit: http://www.partnereartheducationcenter.com/
Currently author of *Plant Spirit Healing* and *Partner Earth*.

18 Grieves M. 1994. *A Modern Herbal*. New York: Dorset Press.

19 Gladstar, Rosemary. 1995. *The Science and Art of Herbalism: Herb Apprentice Course.*

20 Tallamy D. W. 2007. *Bringing Nature Home.* Portland, London: Timber Press.

21 Gladstar, Rosemary. 1995. *The Science and Art of Herbalism: Herb Apprentice Course.*

22 Winston, David. 1989. Class at Green Nations Gathering. Visit: http://www.herbalstudies.net/

23 Grieves M. 1994. *A Modern Herbal.* New York: Dorset Press.

24 Duke, James. A. Ph.D. 1997. *The Green Pharmacy.* Pennsylvania: Rodale Press.

25 Chodron, Pema. *Compassionate Listening* in audio interview. Visit: http://pemachodronfoundation.org/

26 Dawson, Adele, G. 2000. *Herbs: Partners in Life.* Rochester Vermont: Healing Arts Press.

27 Garrett J.T. 2003. *The Cherokee Herbal.* Rochester, Vermont: Bear & Company.

28 Gladstar, Rosemary. 1995. *The Science and Art of Herbalism: Herb Apprentice Course.*

29 Gibbons E. 1966. *Stalking the Healthful Herbs.* New York: David McKay Company, Inc.

30 Myss, Caroline. 2002. *Sacred Contracts.* New York: Three Rivers Press. P. 123-134.

Archetype defined: An inherited idea or mode of thought in the psychology of C.G. Jung that is derived from the experience of the race and is present in the unconscious of the individual.

31 Garrett J.T. 2003. *The Cherokee Herbal.* Rochester, Vermont: Bear & Company.

32 Moss, Robert. 1996. *Conscious Dreaming.* New York: Three Rivers Press.

33 Horvilleur, Alain, MD. 1989. *The Family Guide to Homeopathy*. Virginia, US: Health & Homeopathy Publishing, Inc.

34 Duke, James. 1997. A. Ph.D. *The Green Pharmacy*. Pennsylvania: Rodale Press.

Hoffmann D. 1983. *The Holistic Herbal*. Longmead, Shaftesbury, Dorset: Element Books Ltd.

35 Lad, Vassant. 2002. *Textbook of Ayurveda: Fundamental Principles*. Albuquerque, New Mexico: The Ayurvedic Press.

36 Grieves M. 1994. *A Modern Herbal*. New York: Dorset Press.

37 "The Findhorn Garden Story", 4th edition, by the Findhorn Community © 1975 by the Findhorn Foundation; published by Findhorn Press, Scotland Findhorn Community.

38 Jacke D. with E. Toensmeier. 2005. *Edible Forest Gardens Vol. 1: Ecological Vision and Theory for Temperate Climate Permaculture*. White River Junction, Vermont: Chelsea Green Publishing Company.

39 Roads M. J. 2011. *Conscious Gardening*. Scotland, United Kingdoms: Findhorn Press.

40 Roads M. J. 2011. *Conscious Gardening*. Scotland, United Kingdoms: Findhorn Press.

41 http://healthychild.org/how-pesticides-harm-childrens-health-and-brains

42 http://www.paladinoandco.com/wp-content/uploads/2012/11/Pesticide-FreeCampuses.pd

43 https://edibleschoolyard.org/

44 http://people.csail.mit.edu/seneff/Entropy/entropy-15-01416.pdf

45 Documentary: *Queen of the Sun*.

46 http://www.organicconsumers.org/articles/article_29295.cfm

47 http://people.csail.mit.edu/seneff/

48 http://www.panna.org/science/myths

Other References

Herbs, Plants and Nature

Duke, James. A. Ph.D. 1997. *The Green Pharmacy*. Pennsylvania: Rodale Press.

Foster S. and J.A. Duke 1998. *Eastern/Central Medicinal Plants*. Boston, New York: Houghton Mifflin Company.

Garrett J.T. 2003. *The Cherokee Herbal*. Rochester, Vermont: Bear & Company.

Gibbons E. 1966. *Stalking the Healthful Herbs*. New York: David McKay Company, Inc.

Gibbons E. 1962. *Stalking the Wild Asparagus*. New York: David McKay Company, Inc.

Gladstar R. with Hirsch, P. 2000. *Planting the Future: Saving Our Medicinal Herbs*. Rochester, Vermont: Healing Arts Press.

Grieves M. 1994. *A Modern Herbal*. New York: Dorset Press.

Jacke D. with E. Toensmeier. 2005. *Edible Forest Gardens Vol. 1: Ecological Vision and Theory for Temperate Climate Permaculture*. White River Junction, Vermont: Chelsea Green Publishing Company.

Hoffmann D. 1983. *The Holistic Herbal*. Longmead, Shaftesbury, Dorset: Element Books Ltd.

Hutchens A.R. 1991. *Indian Herbology of North America*. Boston, Massachusetts: Shambhala Publications, Inc.

Martin L. C. 1986. *The Wildflower Meadow Book: A Gardner's Guide*. Old Saybrook, Connecticut.

Newcomb L. 1977. *Newcomb's Wildflower Guide*. Boston-New York-Toronto-London: Little, Brown and Company.

Roads M. J. 2011. *Conscious Gardening*. Scotland, United Kingdoms: Findhorn Press.

Silverman M. 1997. *A City Herbal*. Woodstock, New York: Ash Tree Publishing.

Tallamy D. W. 2007. *Bringing Nature Home*. Portland, London: Timber Press.

Verner Y.1998. *The Blooming Lawn*. White River Junction, Vermont: Chelsea Green Publishing Company.

Native Americans

Arguelles, Jose 1987. *The Mayan Factor*. Santa FE, New Mexico: Sun Bear & Co.

Bear S., Mulligan C., Nufer P., and Wabun. 1989. *Walking in Balance*. New York, New York: Prentice Hall Press.

Bear S. and Wabun. 1980. *The Medicine Wheel*. New York, New York: Prentice Hall Press.

Caduto M. J. and Bruchac J. 1994. *Keepers of Life*. Golden, Colorado: Fulcrum Publishing.

Carter F.1976. *The Education of the Little Tree*. University of New Mexico Press.

Foster S. with Little M. 1962. *The Book of the Vision Quest*. New York: Prentice Hall Press.

Garrett J.T. and Garrett M. 1996. *Medicine of the Cherokee*. Rochester, Vermont; Bear & Company.

Lake-Thom Bobby. 2001. *Call of the Great Spirit*. Rochester, Vermont: Bear & Company.

Mehl-Madrona L. M.D. 1997. *Coyote Medicine*. New York, New York: Scribner.

Millman Dan. 1991. *Sacred Journey of the Peaceful Warrior*. Tiburon, California.

Ross, Dr. A.C. 1998. *Mitakuye Oyasin: "We are all related."* Denver Colorado. Wiconi Waste.

Sams J. and Nitsch T.1991. *Other Council Fires Were Here Before Ours*. San Francisco, California: Harper, San Francisco.

Sams J. 1993. *The 13 Original Clan Mothers*. San Francisco, California: Harper, San Francisco.

Schaffer C. 2006. *Grandmothers Counsel the World*. Boston: Trumpeter Books.

Weatherford J.1991. *Native Roots*. New York: Ballantine Books.

Wolf B. H. 1982. *The Ways of My Grandmothers*. New York: Quill.

Mysticism, Spirituality

Dyer, Dr. Wayne. *The Power of Intention*. United States: Hay House.

Estes, Clarissa Pinkola. 1992. *Women Who Run With the Wolves.* New York: Ballantine books. P. 236-237.

Faraday, Ann. 1990. *The Dream Game.* New York: Harper & Row.

Garfield, Patricia. *Creative Dreaming.* 1976. New York: Ballantine Books.

Moore T. 1992. *Care of the Soul.* New York, New York: HarperCollins Publishers, Inc.

Moore T. 2008. *A Life at Work.* New York: Broadway Books.

Moss, Robert. 1996. *Conscious Dreaming.* New York, New York: Three Rivers Press.

Myss C. 2002. *Sacred Contracts.* New York, New York: Three Rivers Press.

O'Donohue J. 1998. *Anam Cara.* New York, New York: HarperCollins Publishers.

ACKNOWLEDGEMENTS

THIS BOOK RELATES A LEARNING ODYSSEY OVER SEVERAL YEARS. I WISH TO GIVE heartfelt thanks to family and friends who supported me along the way.

To Maka Nupa L Cota: For your support and encouragement to delve deeper while walking a wheel of truths helped me birth this book into being. I honor you and the gift of your friendship.

To Grandmother Twylah, Grandmother Kitty, and my elder brother Toe: You who have passed on, shared much. I honor you.

To my herbal teachers, especially Pam Montgomery who showed me a beginning and to Rosemary Gladstar for her inspiration and knowledge. To fellow herbalists who have always been an inspiration, I give my thanks.

To Sharon McCamy for her wonderful edits so this manuscript could take a polished form. I will be forever grateful.

To Linda Silk for her artistic vision and creating a book cover that speaks to my walk. Thank you.

To my dear sons who played in this meadow and grew into outstanding men: You drank the teas, used the salves; today with your gifts, talents, and patience you help me walk through new gates of understanding. You are the blessings of my life.

To my Mother, who knows the truth of my journey: I honor you and am so grateful for all we have shared together on this path called life.

To those of you I call friend: I thank you for listening, for support, and most important for believing in me. All of you made this journey sparkle.

Last but not least, the Nature Intelligences who guided me and continue to guide me on this earth walk. I hope and pray we can build strong bridges of understanding and cooperation.

To my new friends at FriesenPress, especially Dana Mills and team, I am grateful for your guidance and assistance in making this dream come true.

Namaste everyone.

About The Author

Judith Dreyer, MS, BSN, is a Master Gardener and teacher with over 20 years' experience developing workshops and classes, speaking and writing about holistic health, edible and medicinal plants, dreams and more. She has degrees in Nursing and Nutrition Science and has taught Holistic Health Studies and Nutrition Science at both university and college level.

Judith has traveled a wheel of diverse learning and experiences. Visit her blog. *At the Garden's Gate*: go to: judithdreyer.com

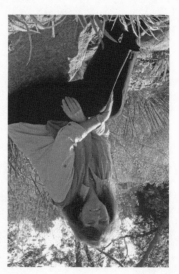